Clinical Management of Cardiovascular Risk Factors in Diabetes

W9-AXE-394

Fourth Edition

Marvin Moser, MD, FACP
Clinical Professor of Medicine
Yale University School of Medicine

James R. Sowers, MD
Professor of Medicine, Physiology,
and Pharmacology
University of Missouri–Columbia

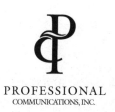

PROFESSIONAL
COMMUNICATIONS, INC.

Professional Communications, Inc.

A Medical Publishing Company

400 Center Bay Drive
West Islip, NY 11795
(t) 631/661-2852
(f) 631/661-2167

PO Box 10
Caddo, OK 74729-0010
(t) 580/367-9838
(f) 580/367-9989

For orders only, please call
1-800-337-9838
or visit our website at
www.pcibooks.com

ISBN: 978-1-932610-62-8

Printed in the United States of America

DISCLAIMER
The opinions expressed in this publication reflect those of the authors. However, the authors make no warranty regarding the contents of the publication. The protocols described herein are general and may not apply to a specific patient. Any product mentioned in this publication should be taken in accordance with the prescribing information provided by the manufacturer.

This text is printed on recycled paper.

DEDICATION

To our colleagues and students who are working to reduce the cardiovascular consequences of diabetes, hypertension, and dyslipidemia. In this era of interventional and procedure-driven medicine, it is important to remember the important contributions that good patient care and attention to risk-factor modification can play in preventing cardiovascular disease.

ACKNOWLEDGMENT

We express our gratitude to Adrienne Cramer, who has worked as a research and administrative assistant to Marvin Moser for many years, and to Malcolm Beasley and Phyllis Freeny for their guidance and help in editing the manuscript. Finally, our thanks to the Hypertension Education Foundation, Inc. for research support.

TABLE OF CONTENTS

TABLES

vii

FIGURES

xi

Preface to Fourth Edition

The prevalence of both diabetes and hypertension are on the increase in the United States, in part related to the increasing incidence of obesity and the aging of our population. Some of the reported increase in diabetes prevalence, however, may also be the result of newer definitions of the disease (ie, change from a fasting blood glucose [FBG] of >140 mg/dL to >126 mg/dL). The coexistence of diabetes and hypertension is also increasingly common, and patients with both disorders are at a considerably higher risk for cardiovascular disease (CVD) than individuals with either disease alone. The fourth edition of *Clinical Management of Cardiovascular Risk Factors in Diabetes* updates current knowledge and guidelines in the prevention and treatment of CVD in patients with coexisting diabetes and hypertension. In addition, it reviews newer data on the management of dyslipidemia and nephropathy in diabetic patients. A clear message emerges—several major risk factors that adversely impact the life of patients with hypertension and/or diabetes can be controlled and lives prolonged if these are controlled. A dramatic decrease in cardiovascular (CV) morbidity and mortality has occurred as a result of better and earlier treatment.

1 Introduction

The history of the prevention of heart attack, stroke, and heart failure by altering known CV risk factors is an exciting one. Perhaps nowhere else has such an impact been made in preventive medicine other than in the prevention of infectious diseases, such as typhoid fever and polio, by the use of vaccines. Interventions to prevent vascular diseases followed the recognition of various factors that increase the risk for CVD. These include hypertension, smoking, and hyperlipidemia. A disease that appears to cluster with many of these factors is diabetes. Most diabetic patients:

- Have elevated blood pressure (BP)
- Are obese
- Have hyperlipidemia
- Have coagulation disorders.

Any one of these specific entities poses a risk for an increase in CV events. When these risk factors occur in conjunction with diabetes, CVD risk is considerably increased.

Until recent years, most efforts in managing diabetes concentrated on glycemic control with diet, insulin, or antidiabetic medications. Most of the studies designed to show that tight control of blood glucose levels would reduce CV events in type 2 diabetic patients have proven to be only marginally successful. With extremely tight glycemic control, some success has been noted in preventing the microvascular complications of diabetes (ie, retinopathy, neuropathy, renal disease, etc), but effects on CV end points have not been consistently demonstrated. One recent study suggests that overly vigorous attempts to reduce blood glucose levels may actually be harmful. This has not been confirmed.

Too many diabetic patients are unable or unwilling to alter their lifestyle enough or to take the appropriate medication to bring about the degree of blood glucose control required to prevent complications. In addition, there are problems with weight gain and hypoglycemic episodes with very tight glycemic control. More attention is focused on interventions to control the other risk factors that occur in the diabetic: The bottom line is that controlling hyperglycemia should only be one part of the effort of a multifaceted approach to reduce vascular complications in diabetic patients.

Hypertension, defined as a persistent BP >140/90 mm Hg, is common in diabetics. It is well recognized that the presence of hypertension in a diabetic patient greatly increases risk not only for CVD but for eye disease and renal failure. It has been known for years that a diabetic patient is at much greater risk for coronary heart disease (CHD) events than a nondiabetic with similar BP. Yet, until recently, careful management of elevated BP has not been emphasized.

The effort to control hypertension has been hindered by a variety of myths and misconceptions. Some of these relate to the following:

- Preoccupation with protecting the kidneys in patients with diabetes. It is recognized that diabetic nephropathy is common and that end-stage renal disease (ESRD) is a fairly frequent and serious outcome in diabetic patients. But most of the deaths that occur prematurely in diabetic patients are secondary to CVD and not renal failure. Treatment to prevent renal disease is of great importance, but as much or more emphasis should be placed on CV outcomes.

- The fact that doubt had been placed in the mind of many physicians about the potential theoretic hazards associated with the use of various antihypertensive drugs, most specifically, diuretics. These agents were, until recent years, the antihypertensive medications used as initial therapy in almost all of the hypertension-treatment clinical trials. Despite the fact that they were effective antihypertensive agents and that their use reduced morbidity and mortality, there were still many physicians who were reluctant to use them because of concerns about possible changes in insulin resistance, blood glucose, lipid levels, and the occurrence of new-onset (incipient) diabetes (NOD).

- Debates about the appropriate BP level at which treatment should be started.
- Concerns about the target to which BP should be lowered. This also delayed a more aggressive approach to the management of hypertension in the patient with diabetes.

Many of these misconceptions have been clarified by results of clinical trials. The trials have shown that lowering of BP in diabetic patients, especially in those with non–insulin-dependent (type 2), will reduce CV events, stroke, and progression of renal disease to a greater degree than the control of elevated blood glucose levels.

This is not to conclude that glycemic control is not important—it is to emphasize that treatment programs focused only on glycemic control in such patients are no longer appropriate. All classes of currently available antihypertensive agents are safe and effective in this population. There are some outcome differences, however, which will be discussed and some preferences for specific therapy.

Treatment with lifestyle modifications and antihypertensive medications should be started earlier in a diabetic hypertensive patient than in a nondiabetic and pursued to BP levels lower than those in the nondiabetic, ie, to levels <130/80 mm Hg (see *Chapter 4* and *Chapter 5*). Data suggest that the lowest risk is associated with a systolic BP (SBP) ≤120 mm Hg. Not only does BP control reduce macrovascular complications (eg, coronary events, heart failure, and stroke), but also microvascular events (eg, retinopathy and proteinuria). As this evidence has emerged from numerous trials, as well as evidence that controlling lipid levels in the diabetic patient is also beneficial, more emphasis has been placed on evaluating the diabetic patient as a panoply of the metabolic and CVD states wrapped in a diagnosis of diabetes. The conglomerate includes hyperglycemia, hyperlipidemia, hypertension, and enhanced coagulation.

Diabetes is a common disease, occurring in approximately 10% of adults in the United States. Hypertension is even more common; >50% of people >55 years of age have elevated BP defined as >140/90 mm Hg. Hyperlipidemia and obesity are present in >40% of adults in the United States.

Numerous textbooks and monographs have been written about the management of hypertension and hyperlipidemia. There are many books dealing with the dietary and drug management of the diabetic individual. *Clinical Management of Cardiovascular Risk Factors in Diabetes* summarizes available data and outlines a practical approach to the management of all of the CV risk factors in an individual with diabetes. The fourth edition updates recent trials, outcome studies, and guidelines that confirm a multifaceted approach to reduce CVD in this high-risk population. It is appropriate to do this so that health care providers may approach the diabetic patient not only as someone in need of dietary guidance, antidiabetic drugs, insulin, or other medications to control blood glucose levels, but as a patient with a complex of factors that can be treated with the expectation that morbidity/mortality will be significantly reduced.

Additional data from prospective, randomized clinical trials are available so that even more specific recommendations can be made than 2 to 3 years ago. These trials continue to demonstrate the benefits of antihypertensive, antiplatelet, and antilipid therapy in diabetic patients. Many of the misconceptions that have limited the use of therapeutic agents in hypertension have been put to rest.

Specific problems relating to hypertensive diabetic patients that may influence the choices of therapy are discussed in *Clinical Management of Cardiovascular Risk Factors in Diabetes*. These unique issues include the facts that diabetic patients often:

- Present with postural hypotension secondary to autonomic neuropathy
- Have a relatively high incidence of sexual dysfunction
- Have subclinical evidence of renal disease, ie, low levels of proteinuria
- Experience "silent" myocardial infarctions (MIs) and a high incidence of subclinical CVD.

Clinical Management of Cardiovascular Risk Factors in Diabetes is not intended to be a textbook. It is intended to:

- Update data on the pathophysiology of diabetes, especially as these relate to part of a clinical syndrome
- Review the specific treatments of elevated blood glucose levels, dyslipidemia, elevated BP, and coagulation abnormalities in the diabetic patient
- Summarize recent and older clinical trials that have established benefits of treatment
- Present a specific outline of treatment recommendations for the diabetic patient with or without some of the other comorbid conditions. This book presents the practitioner with a guideline based on firm scientific evidence. Special problems will be discussed in some detail with specific suggestions as to how they should be handled in the typical diabetic patient.

This fourth edition reviews recent trials and new guidelines and how they can be implemented by the practicing physician.

An optimistic picture can be painted for most patients with diabetes, whether they have type 1 diabetes, a disease that once was almost universally fatal by 35 to 40 years of age, or type 2 diabetes, which often does not manifest itself until the patient is middle-aged or older. Type 1 diabetics live longer and less-confining lives with modern therapy; individuals with type 2 diabetes can now look forward to a life with considerably less fear of morbid events, such as stroke and heart failure, that were once almost expected outcomes. Serious nephropathy and retinopathy can also be delayed or possibly prevented. These events may still occur, but with rigorous treatment of hypertension and hyperlipidemia, as well as of diabetes, they are considerably less common. The earlier the diabetic patient is treated, the greater the chance of preventing CV events.

It is our aim that this book will give the reader a guide to the clinical management of CV risk factors in diabetic patients.

2

Diabetes in the United States

Prevalence and Trends

Diabetes is a metabolic disease characterized by hyperglycemia resulting from defects in insulin action, insulin secretion, or both. As of 2007, 23.6 million Americans had diabetes, representing 7% of the total population. Of those, 90% to 95% have type 2 diabetes. Approximately 6 million Americans may have this metabolic disorder but have not currently been diagnosed. The prevalence is especially high in black and Hispanic persons.

It is predicted that the number of diabetics will increase to 30.3 million Americans and to 366 million people worldwide by 2030 (**Figure 2.1**). Diabetes is more prevalent with increasing age, affecting 2.6% of people aged 20 to 39 years, 10.8% of those 40 to 59 years, but 23.1% of those ≥60 years of age (**Figure 2.2**). This increase in the prevalence of diabetes is primarily due to changing population demographics, including:

- Increasing obesity
- Sedentary lifestyle
- An aging population with a growing percentage of minority populations with a disproportionately high prevalence of diabetes (in the United States) (**Figure 2.3**).

Some of the increased prevalence may, however, be related to the change in definition several years ago from a fasting serum glucose level of >140 mg/dL to a level of 126 mg/dL.

The chronic hyperglycemia of diabetes is associated with long-term vascular damage or dysfunction and the failure of various organs, especially the heart, brain, kidneys, eyes, and nerves (**Figure 2.4**). Untreated diabetes markedly decreases the life span of both men and women (**Figure 2.5**). Health care costs to treat complications related to diabetes exceed $300 billion annually.

21

FIGURE 2.1 — Estimated Number of Adults Worldwide With Diabetes by Age Group and Year

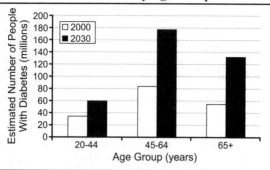

Wild S, et al. *Diabetes Care*. 2004;27:1047-1053.

Diabetes-related complications will increasingly consume a disproportionate share of health care resources unless vigorous efforts are made to control them.

Development of Diabetes

It is clear that our aging population, our increasing minority population (especially Hispanics), and the increase in obesity now seen in a high percentage of children will result in striking increases in the prevalence of type 2 diabetes in the United States over the next decade. The current epidemic of obesity (**Figure 2.6**) is probably the single biggest factor in the great increase in type 2 diabetes that is occurring worldwide (**Figure 2.1**).

Several pathophysiologic abnormalities are involved in the development of diabetes. These vary from autoimmune destruction of the β-cells of the pancreas (type 1 diabetes) with consequent insulin deficiency to abnormalities that result in resistance to the actions of insulin (type 2). The majority of cases of diabetes fall into two broad pathogenetic categories. In one category (type 1 diabetes), the cause is an absolute deficiency of insulin secretion. Persons at increased risk for developing this type of diabetes can often be identified by serologic evidence of an autoimmune pathologic process occurring in the pancreatic islets and by genetic markers. Most often, however, patients are identified when symptoms occur,

FIGURE 2.2 — Estimated Prevalence of Diagnosed and Undiagnosed Diabetes in People Aged ≥20 Years by Age Group: United States, 2007

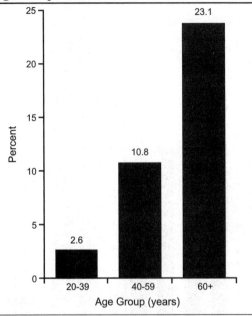

2003-2006 National Health and Nutrition Examination Survey estimates of total prevalence (both diagnosed and undiagnosed) were projected to year 2007.

National Diabetes Statistics, 2007. National Diabetes Information Clearinghouse Web site. http://diabetes.niddk.nih.gov/dm/pubs/statis tics/DM_Statistics.pdf. Accessed November 5, 2009.

such as polyuria, thirst, weight loss, dryness and itching of the skin, etc. In the much more prevalent category (type 2 diabetes), the cause is usually a combination of resistance to insulin action and an inadequate compensatory β-cell insulin secretory response.

In the latter category (>90% of diabetics in the United States), subtle hyperglycemia sufficient to cause pathologic and functional changes in target tissues, but without clinical symptoms, may exist for a long period of time before clinical diabetes is diagnosed. In other words, such patients may actually secrete an excess

FIGURE 2.3 — Estimated Age-Adjusted Total Prevalence of Diabetes in People Aged ≥20 Years by Race/Ethnicity: United States, 2005

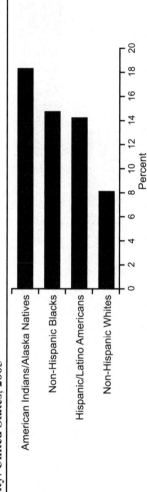

For American Indians/Alaska natives, the estimate of total prevalence was calculated using the estimate of diagnosed diabetes from the 2003 outpatient database of the Indian Health Service and the estimate of undiagnosed diabetes from the 1999-2002 National Health and Nutrition Examination Survey (NHANES). For the other groups, 1999-2002 NHANES estimates of total prevalence (both diagnosed and undiagnosed) were projected to year 2005.

CDC National Diabetes Fact Sheet. CDC Web site. http://www.cdc.gov/diabetes/pubs/estimates05.htm. Accessed November 5, 2009.

FIGURE 2.4 — United Kingdom Prospective Diabetes Study: Epidemiology

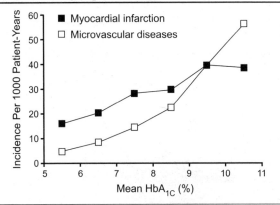

Incidence of both myocardial infarction and microvascular diseases (proteinuria and retinopathy) increases as HbA_{1C} increases. New definitions indicate that a level >7% requires aggressive therapy.

Stratton IM, et al. *BMJ.* 2000;321:405-412.

FIGURE 2.5 — Diabetes Reduces Years of Life

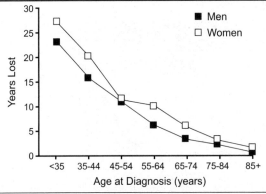

The presence of diabetes markedly reduces life span. For example, a 45- to 54-year old man or woman diagnosed as a diabetic has a life expectancy 10 years less than a nondiabetic (this may have changed recently with more effective therapy for diabetes and comorbid conditions).

Morgan CL, et al. *Diabetes Care.* 2000;23:1103.

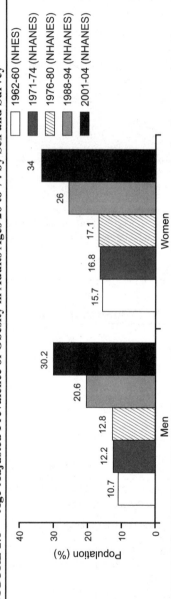

FIGURE 2.6 — Age-Adjusted Prevalence of Obesity in Adults Ages 20 to 74 by Sex and Survey

1962-60 (NHES)
1971-74 (NHANES)
1976-80 (NHANES)
1988-94 (NHANES)
2001-04 (NHANES)

Women
34
26
17.1
16.8
15.7

Men
30.2
20.6
12.8
12.2
10.7

Population (%)

Health, United States, 2006; Unpublished data, NCHS. American Heart Association Web site. http://www.americanheart.org. Accessed May 31, 2007.

amount of insulin for many years but peripheral utilization is decreased, ie, there is increased insulin resistance and blood glucose levels will be at high normal (up to 126 mg/dL fasting). Eventually, the pancreas is unable to keep up with the demand for extra insulin. During this asymptomatic period, it is often possible to demonstrate an abnormality in carbohydrate metabolism by finding elevated plasma glucose or insulin levels following an oral glucose load. This functional abnormality of impaired glucose tolerance (IGT) is often a precursor to clinical type 2 diabetes.

Approximately 10% of Americans have IGT and are at risk for the development of clinical diabetes. Risk factors for progression from IGT include:

- Obesity (**Table 2.1** and **Figure 2.6**)
- Hypertension
- Limited physical activity
- Certain medications (ie, steroids)
- Aging.

TABLE 2.1 — Metabolic and Cardiovascular Risk Factors Associated With Visceral Obesity

- Insulin resistance
- Hyperinsulinemia
- Low high-density lipoprotein cholesterol
- High triglyceride concentrations
- Increased Apo B concentrations
- Increased fibrinogen concentrations
- Increased plasminogen activator
- Increased inhibitor C-reactive protein
- Increased SBP and DBP
- Increased blood viscosity
- Increased left ventricular muscle mass
- Premature atherosclerosis (CHD and stroke)
- Microalbuminuria
- Loss of nocturnal reductions in BP and heart rates

There is also a genetic component to diabetes; the development of the disease is more common when there are close relatives with diabetes and in certain minority populations, such as blacks, Native Americans, and Hispanics. However, it appears that socioeconomic factors, including diet and inactivity, play a role in the higher prevalence of diabetes in these minority populations. People displaying a clinical syndrome of central or abdominal obesity (waist measurement >40 inches in men and >34 inches in women), hypertension, insulin resistance/IGT, hypercoagulability, microalbuminuria, and dyslipidemia have an increased likelihood of developing clinical diabetes. Suggested criteria for testing populations who are at high risk for clinical diabetes are shown in **Table 2.2**.

Type 2 diabetes is frequently not diagnosed until complications appear; many of these patients will have underlying CV disease at the time the diagnosis of diabetes is made. Although the diagnosis of type 2 diabetes increases with advancing age, it is increasingly being

TABLE 2.2 — Criteria for Testing for Prediabetes and Diabetes in Asymptomatic Adult Individuals

- Testing should be considered in all adults who are overweight (BMI $\geq$25 kg/m^2 [a]) and have additional risk factors:
  - Physical inactivity
  - First-degree relative with diabetes
  - Members of a high-risk ethnic population (eg, African American, Latino, Native American, Asian American, Pacific Islander)
  - Women who delivered a baby weighing >9 lb or were diagnosed with GDM
  - Hypertension ($\geq$140/90 mmHg or on therapy for hypertension)
  - HDL cholesterol level <35 mg/dL (0.90 mmol/L) and/or a triglyceride level >250 mg/dL (2.82 mmol/L)
  - Women with polycystic ovarian syndrome
  - IGT or IFG on previous testing
  - Other clinical conditions associated with insulin resistance (eg, severe obesity, acanthosis nigricans)
  - History of CVD
- In the absence of the above criteria, testing for prediabetes and diabetes should begin at age 45 years
- If results are normal, testing should be repeated at least at 3-year intervals, with consideration of more frequent testing depending on initial results and risk status

[a] At-risk BMI may be lower in some ethnic groups.

American Diabetes Association. *Diabetes Care*. 2009;32(suppl 1):S13-S61.

discovered in younger persons, including children and adolescents. The increasing rates of type 2 diabetes in children and adults parallel the increase in overweight (body mass index [BMI] of 25 to 30 kg/m²) and obese (BMI >30 kg/m²) individuals in the United States. Several lifestyle prevention studies have demonstrated the effectiveness of lifestyle modifications, namely, diet and exercise, in the prevention of type 2 diabetes. There is also evidence that angiotensin-converting enzyme (ACE) inhibitors, angiotensin II receptor blockers (ARBs), metformin, thiazolidinediones, and the α-glucosidase inhibitor acarbose can decrease or slow the rate of the development of type 2 diabetes in predisposed persons. One study indicated, however, that while the use of an ACE inhibitor did not prevent the occurrence of diabetes to a statistically significant extent, the use of an antidiabetic agent rosiglitazone was effective.

Diagnostic Criteria for Diabetes

The diagnosis of diabetes mellitus (DM) can be made in three ways as shown in **Table 2.3**, and each should be confirmed at another time by any one of these three methods. The first would include symptoms of diabetes, plus a casual (nonfasting) plasma glucose concentration ≥200 mg/dL. A second would be that of a fasting glucose ≥126 mg/dL, and the third diagnostic criterion would be a 2-hour postprandial or postglucose load of ≥200 mg/dL. Accordingly, the presence of symptoms with a casual plasma glucose of ≥200 mg/dL, confirmed on another day by a fasting plasma glucose ≥126 mg/dL or a 2-hour postload glucose ≥200 mg/dL, would confirm a diagnosis of clinical diabetes.

Undiagnosed type 2 diabetes is common in the United States, with estimates that >6 million persons with this disease are currently undiagnosed. Relevant to this issue is the epidemiologic evidence that diabetic retinopathy (most common cause of new blindness in the United States) begins to develop at least 7 years before the clinical diagnosis of type 2 diabetes is made. Patients with undiagnosed diabetes are also at significantly greater risk for ischemic heart disease, stroke, peripheral vascular

TABLE 2.3 — Criteria for the Diagnosis of Diabetes

1. FPG ≥126 mg/dL (7.0 mmol/L). Fasting is defined as no caloric intake for at least 8 hours[a]

   OR

2. Symptoms of hyperglycemia and a casual (random) plasma glucose ≥200 mg/dL (11.1 mmol/L). Casual (random) is defined as any time of day without regard to time since last meal. The classic symptoms of hyperglycemia include:
   - Polyuria
   - Polydipsia
   - Unexplained weight loss.

   OR

3. 2-Hour plasma glucose ≥200 mg/dL (11.1 mmol/L) during an OGTT. The test should be performed as described by the World Health Organization using a glucose load containing the equivalent of 75-g anhydrous glucose dissolved in water.[a]

[a] In the absence of unequivocal hyperglycemia, these criteria should be confirmed by repeat testing on a different day.

American Diabetes Association. *Diabetes Care*. 2009;32(suppl 1):S13-S61.

disease, and diabetic renal disease. Thus it is important to recognize factors that suggest a high risk for diabetes so appropriate screening and treatment can be carried out.

A relationship that has been recently appreciated is the increased prevalence of type 2 diabetes among persons with hepatitis C virus (HCV) infection in the United States. This relationship is especially strong in persons >40 years of age, nonwhites, those with a high BMI, and individuals of lower socioeconomic status. For example, persons ≥40 years of age with HCV infection are more than three times as likely to have type 2 diabetes as those without HCV infection. Since approximately 2.7 million persons in the United States have chronic HCV infection, this represents another high-risk group that should be screened for type 2 diabetes.

Pathogenesis of Type 2 Diabetes

Two major pathophysiologic factors contribute to the development of type 2 diabetes:
- Insulin resistance
- Impaired pancreatic β-cell function.

■ Insulin Resistance

Insulin resistance is relatively common in adults in the United States. Data from the Insulin Resistance Atherosclerosis Study (IRAS) show that 90% of obese blacks, whites, and Hispanic Americans with type 2 diabetes may be classified as insulin insensitive or resistant. Insulin resistance in conjunction with hyperinsulinemia has also been identified more than a decade before the onset of diabetes in the obese offspring of persons with type 2 diabetes.

Insulin resistance is associated with diminished glucose disposal and dyslipidemia. In skeletal muscle, the major tissue involved in glucose disposal, there is deficient insulin-mediated glucose transport with subsequent impairment of oxidation and glycogen storage. In the liver, insulin resistance is associated with reduced postprandial glucose storage and the ability of insulin to inhibit lipolysis to suppress glycogenolysis and gluconeogenesis in the fasting and postprandial states. The ability of insulin to inhibit lipolysis in adipose tissue is also diminished.

Insulin resistance is associated with a group of metabolic and hemodynamic abnormalities known as the cardiometabolic syndrome.

Studies in high-risk populations suggest that the insulin-resistant phenotype, like type 2 diabetes, has a genetic component. To date, however, no specific genetic defect has been found in the majority of patients with type 2 diabetes to explain their metabolic disease solely due to insulin resistance. Environmental factors appear to be the main determinant of insulin resistance.

■ Impaired Pancreatic β-Cell Function

Most patients who are obese and insulin resistant do not develop diabetes. They have the ability to compensate for insulin resistance by increasing insulin secretion. Therefore, the development of type 2 diabetes involves a defect in compensatory insulin secretion.

Possible causes of β-cell dysfunction, the other major causative factor in diabetes, include:

- Amyloid deposition or inflammation/apoptosis or other conditions that reduce β-cell mass
- Sustained insulin resistance leading to β-cell exhaustion
- Glucose and/or lipid toxicity to β-cells
- Autoimmune β-cell destruction.

According to data from the United Kingdom Prospective Diabetes Study (UKPDS), β-cell function was reduced 50% at the time of diagnosis of type 2 diabetes, and there was progressive loss of function over time.

SELECTED READING

American Diabetes Association. Standards of medical care in diabetes. *Diabetes Care*. 2009;32(suppl 1):S13-S61.

Boyle JP, Honeycutt AA, Narayan KM, et al. Projection of diabetes burden through 2050: impact of changing demography and disease prevalence in the U.S. *Diabetes Care*. 2001;24:1936-1940.

Buchanan TA, Xiang AH, Peters RK, et al. Preservation of pancreative beta-cell function and prevention of type 2 diabetes by pharmacological treatment of insulin resistance in high-risk Hispanic women. *Diabetes*. 2002;51:2796-2803.

Chiasson JL, Josse RG, Gomis R, Hanefeld M, Karasik A, Laakso M; STOP-NIDDM Trial Research Group. Acarbose for prevention of type 2 diabetes mellitus: the STOP-NIDDM randomised trial. *Lancet*. 2002;359:2072-2077.

DREAM (Diabetes REduction Assessment with ramipril and rosiglitazone Medication) Trial Investigators, Gerstein HC, Yusuf S, Bosch J, et al. Effect of rosiglitazone on the frequency of diabetes in patients with impaired glucose tolerance or impaired fasting glucose: a randomised controlled trial. *Lancet*. 2006;368:1096-1105.

Gerich JE. Contibutions of insulin-resistance and insulin-secretory defects to the pathogenesis of type 2 diabetes mellitus. *Mayo Clin Proc*. 2003;78:447-456.

Knowler WC, Barrett-Connor E, Fowler SE, et al; Diabetes Prevention Program Research Group. Reduction in the incidence of type 2 diabetes with lifestyle intervention or metformin. *N Engl J Med*. 2002;346:393-403.

Mehta SH, Brancati FL, Sulkowski MS, Strathdee SA, Szklo M, Thomas DL. Prevalence of type 2 diabetes mellitus among persons with hepatitis C virus infection in the United States. *Ann Intern Med*. 2000;133:592-599.

Mokdad AH, Ford ES, Bowman BA, et al. Prevalence of obesity, diabetes, and obesity-related health risk factors, 2001. *JAMA*. 2003;289:76-79.

Sowers JR, Haffner S. Treatment of cardiovascular and renal risk factors in the diabetic hypertensive. *Hypertension*. 2002;40:781-788.

Sowers JR, Lester MA. Diabetes and cardiovascular disease. *Diabetes Care*. 1999;22(suppl 3):C14-C20.

Stratton IM, Adler A, Neil HA, et al. Association of glycaemia with macrovascular and microvascular complications of type 2 diabetes (UKPDS 35): prospective observational study. *BMJ*. 2000;321:405-412.

Tuomilehto J, Lindstrom J, Eriksson JG, et al; Finnish Diabetes Prevention Study Group. Prevention of type 2 diabetes mellitus by changes in lifestyle among subjects with impaired glucose tolerance. *N Engl J Med*. 2001;344:1343-1350.

3

Scope of and Risk Factors for Cardiovascular Disease in Diabetic Patients

Cardiovascular Disease in Diabetics

Whereas CVD accounts for 40% of the overall mortality in the United States, nearly 80% of deaths in type 2 diabetic persons are secondary to complications of CVD, such as:

- Sudden death
- MI
- Congestive heart failure (CHF)
- Cerebrovascular and peripheral vascular disease.

All of the above complications are considerably more common in diabetics than in nondiabetics. Many of these can be reduced by early, effective treatment of diabetes and associated comorbidities.

The risk for CVD mortality is approximately 2-fold in diabetic men and 4-fold in diabetic women when compared with people without diabetes. The relative risk for stroke in persons with diabetes is 2- to 3-fold higher than in nondiabetic persons and is higher in females than in males. The UKPDS group found that over an 8-year period, increased risk for stroke in diabetic persons was related to a diagnosis of hypertension or to higher SBP, regardless of whether BP was measured in treated or untreated persons. Even people with SBP between 125 and 142 mm Hg had twice the risk for stroke observed in persons with lower levels of SBP. Information from death certificates indicates that hypertension is implicated in many of the deaths coded to diabetes and that diabetes is involved in >10% of deaths coded to hypertension-related disease. While much of the attention relating to diabetes treatment has centered on prevention of diabetic nephropathy and ESRD, CVD is far more common as an outcome in this population.

It is important to emphasize that some, but not all, data suggest that a diabetic without a history of MI is at the same risk for a CV event as a nondiabetic patient with a history of an MI (**Figure 3**.1). In other words, any diabetic patient should be considered at high risk for CVD. This reconsideration is important in therapy considerations (see *Chapter 4* and *Chapter 5*).

■ **Cardiovascular Disease in Diabetic Men**
In the Multiple Risk Factor Intervention Trial (MRFIT), >5000 men with diabetes were observed for 12 years and compared with >350,000 men without diabetes. The risk of CVD death at 12 years was 3-fold higher in

FIGURE 3.1 — Risk of Cardiovascular Events in Type 2 Diabetes

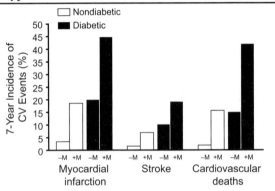

Key: –M, no prior MI; +M, prior MI.

Type 2 diabetes is associated with a marked increase in the risk of CV disease. Seven-year incidences of fatal or nonfatal MI, fatal or nonfatal stroke, and death from CV causes among 1373 nondiabetic subjects were compared with the incidences among 1059 patients with type 2 diabetes. Both the presence of diabetes and the history of a previous MI at baseline were associated with an increased incidence of CV events. In both diabetic patients and nondiabetic subjects, history of prior MI at baseline was significantly associated with an increased incidence of MI, stroke, and CV death. Diabetic patients without prior MI, however, had as high a CV risk as nondiabetic subjects with previous MI.

Haffner SM, et al. *N Engl J Med*. 1998;339:229-234.

diabetic men compared with controls, regardless of age, ethnicity, cholesterol levels, SBP, or tobacco use. Even when patients had optimal SBP and were nonsmokers, the relative risk of CVD death was still 2.5 times higher in those who were diabetic. The MRFIT study underscored the fact that diabetes is a strong independent risk factor for CVD mortality and that systolic hypertension, hypercholesterolemia, and cigarette smoking are also significant independent predictors of mortality in men with and without diabetes. The presence of one or more of these risk factors, in turn, had a significantly greater bearing on CVD risk in the diabetic than in the nondiabetic cohort. The association of an elevated SBP and CV death in diabetics is especially strong (**Figure 3.2**)

FIGURE 3.2 — Association of Systolic Blood Pressure and Cardiovascular Death in Type 2 Diabetes

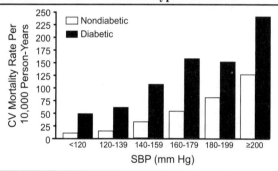

In the Multiple Risk Factor Intervention Trial (MRFIT), the relationships of SBP and other CV risk factors to CV mortality were compared in men with diabetes ($n = 5163$) and without diabetes ($n = 342,815$). The absolute risk of CV death was three times higher for men with diabetes than for those without diabetes. SBP was positively related to the risk of CV death, with a significant trend in both nondiabetic and diabetic subjects ($P < 0.001$). At every level of SBP, however, CV death was much greater in men with diabetes than in men without diabetes. The higher the SBP, the greater the absolute excess risk for patients with diabetes and the greater potential for prevention of CV death among patients with diabetes by control of elevated SBP.

Stamler J, et al. *Diabetes Care.* 1993;16:434-444.

■ Cardiovascular Disease in Diabetic Women

The incidence of CVD increases with increasing age in the United States and other westernized countries, and elderly women constitute a disproportionate component of the aging population. In the United States each year, >240,000 women die from MI and >88,000 die from stroke. For a 50-year-old nondiabetic woman, the lifetime risk of having CHD is 46% and the risk of dying from this disease is now about 30%. Despite a decrease in CHD mortality in most developed countries, the absolute number of CHD deaths in the elderly, particularly in aging diabetic women, has increased.

Population demographics suggest that in the United States, the number of persons >80 years of age in 25 to 30 years will increase dramatically. The number of women in this age group is and will continue to be disproportionately high.

Although CVD is generally less prevalent in premenopausal women than in age-matched men, this difference disappears after menopause, presumably related to decreased estrogen production. In diabetes (type 1 *or* type 2), this gender difference in CVD is not seen in people <50 years of age, probably because the metabolic and hemodynamic benefits of endogenous estradiol are canceled by the diabetic syndrome. Controlled clinical trials underscore the critical importance of aggressively treating CVD risk factors, especially dyslipidemia and hypertension, in women with diabetes. However, hormone replacement therapy (HRT) is not generally indicated for these postmenopausal women, given their marked propensity for hypercoagulability. Data suggest a possible increase in CVD risk with HRT.

CVD, not ESRD, is the leading cause of death in women with diabetes (as it is in men). In the Framingham Heart Study, MI, angina, and sudden death were 2-fold higher in diabetic than in nondiabetic persons. In addition to removing the normal premenopausal CVD protection, diabetes is a greater CVD mortality risk factor in women than in men >50 years of age. Women with diabetes are also more likely to die after an MI than nondiabetic women or men with or without diabetes. The risk of death from CHD in women with diabetes is >3-fold that in nondiabetic women.

Many factors contribute to the increase in CVD in diabetic women as well as in men, including:

- Hypertension
- Lipoprotein abnormalities
- Endothelial dysfunction
- Increased vascular oxidative stress
- Reduced vascular compliance
- Enhanced platelet aggregation/adhesion
- Enhanced coagulation/reduced fibrinolysis.

Microvascular Disease in Diabetes

■ Diabetic Retinopathy

Certain complications are specific to the diabetic patient. Diabetic retinopathy is the most common cause of new blindness in Americans between the ages of 20 and 74 in the United States. In patients with type 2 diabetes, early manifestations of retinopathy (typically microaneurysm) noted as dot or punctate hemorrhages are common within 5 years after diagnosis of diabetes. Up to 90% of these patients will have some evidence of retinopathy by 15 years postdiagnosis. The presence of proliferative retinopathy is progressive over the course of both type 1 and type 2 diabetes.

Type 1 diabetics should be evaluated by an ophthalmologist yearly, starting 5 years after diagnosis of diabetes. Type 2 diabetic patients should have an ophthalmologic evaluation yearly, starting from the time of diagnosis. Because of accelerated disease during pregnancy, ophthalmologic evaluation is recommended during the first trimester, with follow-up throughout pregnancy. Early treatment of hypertension and diabetes will frequently reduce or prevent the retinal complications of diabetes.

Treatment of diabetic retinopathy primarily involves laser photocoagulation. Focal coagulation is done for the destruction of new vessels or treatment of clinically significant macular edema. Panretinal photocoagulation (sparing the macula) is conducted to destroy ischemic retina and decrease the stimulus to neovascularization.

The intent of such therapy is to regress neovascularization and decrease the risk of subsequent hemorrhage. This technique, however, can exacerbate preexisting macular edema, especially if applied too aggressively.

■ Diabetic Neuropathy

Diabetic neuropathy is another specific complication of diabetes. This is most commonly manifested by orthostatic hypotension.

■ Diabetic Nephropathy

Approximately 30% to 35% of persons with type 1 diabetes will develop nephropathy. The likelihood of type 2 patients developing nephropathy is less, but because of the 10-fold greater prevalence of type 2 diabetes, it is the leading cause of ESRD.

The first laboratory abnormality that indicates the development of diabetic nephropathy is the appearance of small quantities of albumin in the urine, microalbuminuria, sometimes referred to as "incipient diabetic nephropathy" (**Table 3.1**). When the level of albumin is measurable by conventional dipstick, it is referred to as clinical albuminuria. This indicates a progressive decrease in the glomerular filtration rate (GFR). The rate of progression from microalbuminuria to clinical albuminuria and the rate of decline in GFR are both modifiable by treatment (see *Chapter 4*). The presence of microalbuminuria has been independently associated with an increased risk of CVD (see *Chapter 4*).

TABLE 3.1 — Definitions of Abnormalities in Albumin Excretion[a]

Category	24-h Collection	Spot Collection
Normal	<30 mg/24 h	<30 mcg/min creatinine
Microalbuminuria	30-300 mg/24 h	30-300 mcg/min creatinine
Clinical albuminuria	>300 mg/24 h	>300 mcg/min creatinine

[a] Screen for albuminuria once a year (dipstick); if negative, check for microalbuminuria (Micral test).

■ **General Treatment Strategies if Microalbuminuria Is Detected**

Several guidelines committees have recommended rigorous glycemic control to decrease the likelihood of the development of microalbuminuria and to delay the progression of microalbuminuria in both type 1 and type 2 patients with preexisting microalbuminuria (see *Chapter 5*, in section entitled *Vascular Health in the Diabetic Patient With Hypertension* and the discussion of the UKPDS).

Early studies from the STENO diabetes center in Denmark showed that even modest control of hypertension with triple-drug therapy (diuretic/β-blocker/vasodilator) can strikingly decrease the decline of GFR in patients with established diabetic nephropathy. These studies established the importance of rigorous BP control, presaging the current recommendation of a treatment goal of <130/80 mm Hg in diabetic patients. The role of ACE inhibitors and ARBs as part of this treatment strategy is discussed in *Chapter 7*.

Cardiovascular Risk Factors

Diabetes itself should be considered an independent risk factor for CVD in men and women. Other major risk factors for CVD in diabetics as well as in other individuals include:

- Smoking
- Elevated BP
- Abnormal serum lipids and lipoproteins.

Hyperglycemia and insulin resistance increase the significance of these risk factors. Other predisposing risk factors for the development of CVD in patients with diabetes include:

- Obesity
- Physical inactivity
- Family history of CVD
- Advancing age.

These are similar to the risk factors contributing to insulin resistance.

■ Smoking as a Risk Factor

Cigarette smoking is the most important preventable cause of illness and premature death in the United States. There is increasing evidence that cigarette smoking has a synergistic effect with diabetes in raising morbidity and mortality in both type 1 and type 2 diabetic patients. Unfortunately, smoking prevalence among diabetic patients has been reported to be approximately the same as in the general population. Several studies have shown that physician counseling during a simple routine consultation increases the likelihood that patients will stop smoking. One study indicates that a structured intervention program conducted by a nurse in both primary care and hospital settings can achieve a significant increase in smoking cessation in diabetics. Thus it is imperative that health care providers emphasize the especially high risk attributable to smoking in diabetic patients and the overall health benefits of smoking cessation. The high baseline risk for CVD within a 10-year period in diabetics should be emphasized in counseling to promote smoking cessation.

■ Interaction Among Risk Factors

The incidence of both DM and essential hypertension increases with advancing age in industrialized, westernized societies. Data from nonindustrialized societies do not demonstrate this striking age-related increase in incidence, underlying the importance of environmental factors, such as obesity and a sedentary lifestyle. In industrialized societies, advancing age is often associated with a loss of lean body mass, particularly that of skeletal muscle tissue and bone. Skeletal muscle is the predominant site of insulin action to promote glucose uptake, and the decrease in skeletal muscle tissue likely contributes to the increasing insulin resistance associated with aging. The loss of lean body mass is also associated with an increase in relative body fat, particularly abdominal fat. Abdominal fat, particularly that known as visceral fat located in the mesenteric/omental region, is pathophysiologically linked to insulin resistance, impaired glucose tolerance, and hypertension (see *Chapter 4*).

■ Metabolic Syndrome

The metabolic syndrome (previously "Syndrome X") characterized by insulin resistance, hypertension, abdominal obesity, hyperglycemia, elevated triglycerides, and low levels of high-density lipoprotein cholesterol is now well recognized as a major CV risk factor. The major clinical features of the metabolic syndrome are listed in **Table 3.2**. It should be noted that the metabolic syndrome is not a disease but rather a cluster of risk factors that increase the risk for CV disease.

Although there are several different definitions of the metabolic syndrome with regard to specific criteria from national guideline committees, there is general agreement regarding the central importance of abdominal obesity and insulin resistance. The association of the metabolic syndrome, even by different criteria, is associated with hazard ratios for CV death ranging from 1.25 to 2.0 in the general population.

TABLE 3.2 — Clinical Features of the Metabolic Syndrome

Risk Factor	Criteria for Risk
Abdominal obesity:	
Men	Waist circumference: ≥40 in (102 cm)[a]
Women	Waist circumference: ≥35 in (88 cm)[a]
Triglycerides	≥150 mg/dL (or receiving specific treatment)
HDL cholesterol:	
Men	<40 mg/dL (or receiving specific treatment)
Women	<50 mg/dL (or receiving specific treatment)
BP	≥130/≥85 mm Hg
Fasting glucose	≥100 mg/dL (or previously diagnosed type 2 diabetes)

Note: Although definitions proposed by groups such as NCEP/ATP III, AHA/NHLBI, and IDF vary slightly in terms of specific criteria, there is general agreement regarding these five risk factors.

[a] US values; these may vary in different populations.

Adapted from: Alberti KG, et al. *Circulation*. 2009;120:1640-1645.

■ Other Biomarkers of Risk

The established CV risk factors, including dyslipidemia, smoking, hypertension, and DM, have been incorporated into algorithms for risk assessment in the general population. In addition to these and other composites such as the metabolic syndrome, there has been substantial interest in the use of possible newer biomarkers to identify ambulatory persons who are at risk for the development of CV. Many individual biomarkers have been related to CV risk including:

- C-reactive protein (CRP)
- B-type natriuretic peptide
- *N*-terminal proatrial natriuretic peptide
- Aldosterone
- Renin
- Fibrinogen
- D-dimer
- Plasminogen-activator inhibitor type 1 (PAI-1)
- Homocysteine
- Urinary albumin-to-creatinine ratio.

It has been proposed that measurement of several such biomarkers simultaneously (the "multimarker" approach) could enhance risk stratification of individuals in the general adult population.

A study evaluated the usefulness of these biomarkers for predicting death and major CV events during median follow up of 7.4 years in a community-based cohort of 3209 participants attending a routine examination cycle of the Framingham Heart Study. Although several of these biomarkers were associated with increased risk of death, the biomarkers that most strongly predicted major CV events were the B-type natriuretic peptide level and the urinary albumin-to-creatinine ratio. The addition of multimarker scores to conventional risk factors (eg, age, BP, lipid levels, etc) resulted in only small increases in the ability to classify risk. The investigators concluded that the use of the studied biomarkers for assessing risk in individual persons added only moderately to the use of standard risk factors. At present, it is probably not necessary to evaluate these markers to establish the level of risk or determine therapy.

SELECTED READING

American Diabetes Association. Standards of medical care in diabetes. *Diabetes Care*. 2009;32(suppl 1):S13-S61.

Bell DS. Stroke in the diabetic patient. *Diabetes Care*. 1994;17:213-219.

Buse JB, Ginsberg HN, Bakris GL, et al; American Heart Association; American Diabetes Association. Primary prevention of cardiovascular diseases in people with diabetes mellitus: a scientific statement from the American Heart Association and the American Diabetes Association. *Diabetes Care*. 2007;30:162-172.

Canga N, De Irala J, Vara E, Duaso MJ, Ferrer A, Martinez-Gonzalez MA. Intervention study for smoking cessation in diabetic patients: a randomized controlled trial in both clinical and primary care settings. *Diabetes Care*. 2000;23:1455-1460.

Davis TM, Millns H, Stratton IM, Holman RR, Turner RC. Risk factors for stroke in type 2 diabetes mellitus: United Kingdom Prospective Diabetes Study (UKPDS) 29. *Arch Intern Med*. 1999;159:1097-1103.

DECODE Study Group. Does diagnosis of the metabolic syndrome detect further men at high risk of cardiovascular death beyond those identified by a conventional cardiovascular risk score? The DECODE Study. *Eur J Cardiovasc Prev Rehabil*. 2007;14:192-199.

de Simone G, Devereux RB, Chinali M, et al. Prognostic impact of metabolic syndrome by different definitions in a population with high prevalence of obesity and diabetes: the Strong Heart Study. *Diabetes Care*. 2007;30:1851-1856.

Haffner SM, Lehto S, Ronnemaa T, Pyorala K, Laakso M. Mortality from coronary heart disease in subjects with type 2 diabetes and in nondiabetic subjects with and without prior myocardial infarction. *N Engl J Med*. 1998;339:229-234.

Haire-Joshu D, Glasgow RE, Tibbs TL. Smoking and diabetes. *Diabetes Care*. 1999;22:1887-1898.

Hypertension in Diabetes Study Group. Hypertension in Diabetes Study (HDS):1. Prevalence of hypertension in newly presenting type 2 diabetic patients and the association with risk factors for cardiovascular and diabetic complications. *J Hypertens*. 1993;11:309-317.

Liu J, Grundy SM, Wang W, et al. Ten-year risk of cardiovascular incidence related to diabetes, prediabetes, and the metabolic syndrome. *Am Heart J*. 2007;153:552-558.

Lorenzo C, Williams K, Hunt KJ, Haffner SM. The National Cholesterol Education Program–Adult Treatment Panel III, International Diabetes Federation, and World Health Organization definitions of the metabolic syndrome as predictors of incident cardiovascular disease and diabetes. *Diabetes Care*. 2007;30:8-13.

Nilsson PM, Engstrom G, Hedblad B. The metabolic syndrome and incidence of cardiovascular disease in non-diabetic subjects-a population-based study comparing three different definitions. *Diabet Med.* 2007;24:464-472.

Noto D, Barbagallo CM, Cefalu AB, et al. The metabolic syndrome predicts cardiovascular events in subjects with normal fasting glucose: results of a 15 year follow-up in a Mediterranean population. *Atherosclerosis.* 2008;197:147-153.

Sowers JR, Epstein M, Frohlich ED. Diabetes, hypertension, and cardiovascular disease: an update. *Hypertension.* 2001;37:1053-1059.

Stratton IM, Adler A, Neil HA, et al. Association of glycaemia with macrovascular and microvascular complications of type 2 diabetes (UKPDS 35): prospective observational study. *BMJ.* 2000;321:405-412.

Wang TJ, Gona P, Larson MG, et al. Multiple biomarkers for the prediction of first major cardiovascular events and death. *N Engl J Med.* 2006;355:2631-2639.

4

Cardio-Renal-Metabolic Interactions Between Diabetes, Cardiometabolic Syndrome, and Cardiovascular and Renal Disease

Obesity, Insulin Resistance, and Hypertension

Insulin resistance and increased abdominal obesity are important components of the cardiometabolic syndrome (**Table 4.1**). As noted, insulin resistance is closely related to visceral or abdominal obesity. Central or visceral adipose tissue is associated with and contributes to systemic inflammation. Central adipose tissue secretes a number of cytokines (adipokines) that contribute to inflammation, insulin resistance, and other components of the cardiometabolic syndrome. Interventions designed to prevent the accumulation of visceral fat (ie, caloric restriction and exercise) have been shown to decrease age-related increases in insulin resistance and IGT. Based on these and other experimental data, it appears that insulin resistance associated with visceral adiposity is caused in part by abnormalities in fatty acid metabolism. Both mesenteric and omental fat are resistant to the actions of insulin. This results in accelerated lipolysis or breakdown of fatty material. The increased release of free fatty acids (FFAs) into the portal blood supply in turn lends to hepatic overproduction of triglycerides and a decrease in the synthesis of high-density lipoprotein (HDL) (characteristic abnormalities seen in both diabetes and hypertension) (**Table 2.1**).

In addition, increased fatty acids tend to increase skeletal muscle resistance to the actions of insulin. This, in turn, leads to a reduced metabolism of triglyceride-rich particles like very low-density lipoprotein (VLDL). Triglycerides are also increased by this mechanism and HDL levels are decreased.

TABLE 4.1 — Definitions of the Cardiometabolic Syndrome

Diagnostic Criteria	NCEP Definition[a]	WHO Definition[b]
Hyperinsulinemia or insulinemia	—	Hyperinsulinemia ($\geq$75% of normal) or insulin resistance (clamp)
Fasting glycemia or OGTT (2-hour)	Fasting glycemia: $\geq$110 mg/dL	Fasting glycemia ($\geq$110 mg/dL) or OGTT (2-hour) $\geq$140 mg/dL
Waist	Waist: $\geq$102 cm (men) $\geq$88 cm (women)	Waist-to-hip ratio: $\geq$0.90 (men) $\geq$0.88 (women), or BMI: $\geq$30 kg/m^2
Triglycerides	$\geq$150 mg/dL	$\geq$150 mg/dL
HDL cholesterol	<40 mg/dL (men) <50 mg/dL (women)	<35 mg/dL (men) <39 mg/dL (women)
BP	$\geq$130/80 mm Hg	$\geq$140/90 mm Hg
Microalbuminuria or urine albumin/ creatinine ratio	—	Microalbuminuria $\geq$20 mg/min or urine albumin/creatinine ratio $\geq$30 mg/g

[a] NCEP definition requires presence of at least three of the diagnostic criteria.
[b] WHO definition requires presence of hyperinsulinemia (fasting insulin in the upper quartiles of normal) of fasting glycemia $\geq$100 mg/dL and at least two of the above diagnostic criteria.

Increased FFA also contributes to impaired vascular endothelial-derived vasodilation. Thus increased FFA represents one of the important links between obesity, insulin resistance, and the development of hypertension, an integral component of the cardiometabolic syndrome in blood pressure (BP) ≥130/85 mm Hg. In addition to elevated levels of FFAs, there is increased ectopic distribution of fat in persons with the cardiometabolic syndrome. Ectopic fat in heart, skeletal muscle, and liver is associated with increased systemic markers of inflammation and oxidative stress, which likely contribute to increased heart, kidney, and vascular disease associated with the cardiometabolic syndrome.

The age-related increase in fat mass is greater in women than in men. There is an acceleration in the accumulation of central adipose tissue that occurs postmenopausally. This increase in visceral adiposity may account for increases in the prevalence of hypertension and diabetes in postmenopausal women. Regularly performed exercise may protect against, but does not abolish, the increase in "fatness" with aging. One investigation showed that even when master athletes maintain optimal exercise intensity and duration, body fat still increased by approximately 27% in people >65 years of age over a 10-year period. Physically active men and women do, however, have less central adiposity than their sedentary counterparts. Exercise-intervention studies have shown that endurance training selectively reduces body fat centrally. These observations are important in that visceral adiposity (as mentioned earlier) is strongly associated with diabetes, hypertension, CVD, and chronic kidney disease (CKD).

Population-based surveys of adults have revealed that as many as 50% of persons with hypertension have glucose intolerance. The majority of hypertensive persons demonstrating this characteristic are overweight or obese. Studies have also demonstrated, however, that even hypertensive persons with normal weight may have impaired glucose metabolism; more insulin is required to handle a glucose load in insulin-resistant than in insulin-sensitive persons. It has been suggested that the insulin resistance and IGT associated with essential hypertension

49

may be due to decreased skeletal muscle blood flow as a result of vasoconstriction or a deficit in insulin-mediated signaling pathways. Finally, because of aging and inactivity, the relative number of insulin-sensitive muscle fibers decrease. These adverse skeletal muscle changes are important as about 70% of insulin-mediated glucose uptake occurs in skeletal muscle tissue. Exercise intervention studies have demonstrated that all of these skeletal muscle abnormalities can be improved through aerobic exercise.

Persons with hypertension display other metabolic abnormalities that are also generally seen in diabetes. As noted, many of them have lower levels of HDL, higher levels of triglycerides and VLDL, and abnormal small, dense, and more atherogenic low-density lipoprotein (LDL) particles (**Table 4.2**) when compared with normotensive individuals of the same age and weight. In addition, factors such as an increase in fibrinogen and PAI-1 that enhance the tendency for clotting and a decrease in fibrinolytic activity (ie, plasminogen activator levels) are present; hence the need for therapy (aspirin) to decrease clotting tendencies and reduce the risk of CVD.

TABLE 4.2 — Lipoprotein Abnormalities in Patients With Hypertension as Well as in Those With Diabetes Mellitus

- Increased plasma levels of:
  - VLDL
  - LDL
  - Lipoprotein (a)
- Decreased plasma HDL cholesterol
- Increased plasma triglyceride levels
- Increased lipoprotein oxidation
- Increased small dense LDL cholesterol products
- Decreased lipoprotein lipase activity

Genetic studies, including parent-child, twin, and gene studies, have yielded data suggesting a genetic basis for the relationship between hypertension and the metabolic abnormalities noted in diabetes. For example, there are higher heritability tendencies in twins compared with nontwin siblings for BP, LDL, VLDL, and BMI changes. Almost 70% of adults with hypertension before age 55 years have siblings or parents with hypertension, and 12% of all hypertensive persons have dyslipidemia as well as hypertension. Thus both hypertension and diabetes have some genetic basis, and both conditions have been linked to insulin resistance. It is not a given, however, that if there is diabetes with hypertension in the family, offspring will necessarily inherit these conditions.

In addition to the well-recognized relationship between the cardiometabolic syndrome and the future development of type 2 diabetes and hypertension, a number of studies have established a relationship between obesity and other components of the cardiometabolic syndrome and progressive renal failure (**Figure 4.1**). There is an estimated >9 million Americans with CKD (estimated GFR of ≤60 mL/minutes).

Hypertension and Diabetes

Persons with hypertension are at least twice as likely as normotensives to progress to clinical diabetes over a 5-year period, regardless of whether they receive antihypertensive drug therapy. In the early stages of insulin resistance, there is a compensatory increase in insulin secretion and concentration. Over time, pancreatic secretion of insulin decreases and a state of relative deficit of insulin occurs, leading to type 2 diabetes. Insulin normally causes vasodilation in the peripheral vessels. However, when there is insulin resistance as in diabetes and hypertension, there is an impaired vasodilatory response to insulin. Thus insulin resistance may contribute to increased vascular resistance as well as to impaired glucose uptake in insulin-sensitive tissues, such as fat and skeletal muscle.

Studies (eg, Heart Outcomes Prevention Evaluation [HOPE], Valsartan Antihypertensive Long-term Use Evaluation [VALUE], and Antihypertensive and Lipid-Lowering Treatment to Prevent Heart Attack Trial [ALLHAT]) suggest that fewer hypertensive patients develop type 2 diabetes with the use of an ACE inhibition or the use of an ARB compared with regimens that do not include these agents. CHD outcome, however, was not

FIGURE 4.1 — Relationship Between Obesity and Insulin Resistance/Compensatory Hyperinsulinemia, Components of the Metabolic Syndrome, and the Development of Renal Injury, Chronic Kidney Disease, End-Stage Renal Disease, and Cardiovascular Disease

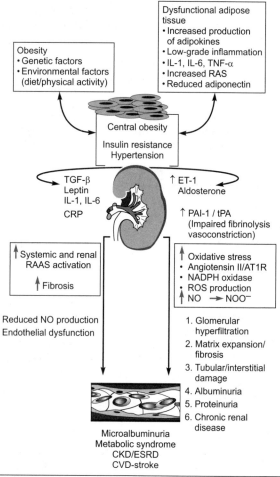

Insulin resistance and compensatory hyperinsulinemia are at the root of activation of the RAS, oxidative stress, low-chronic systemic inflammation, glomerular hypertension, microalbuminura, matrix expansion, and fibrosis.

affected by the difference in NOD among drugs in the double-blind ALLHAT study after 5 years. Insulin resistance in patients with hypertension may also be related to alterations in blood flow to skeletal muscle (**Figure 4.2**). However, in the Diabetes Reduction Assessment With Ramipril and Rosiglitazone Medication (DREAM) trial, ramipril did not demonstrate a diabetes prevention effect but was associated with an increased rate of conversion from impaired fasting and glucose tolerance to normoglycemia in prediabetics. This suggests that RAAS inhibition does have beneficial effects on insulin-mediated glucose utilization.

As previously noted, in hypertensive persons, particularly those who are sedentary, there may be a preponderance of insulin-resistant type II muscle fibers. In contrast, active normotensive persons have relatively more type I skeletal muscle fibers that are insulin sensitive. Thus agents that increase nutrient delivery to skeletal muscle tissues (ie, ACE inhibitors) or other vasodilators (through effects on small vessels) and exercise (through increasing insulin-sensitive red muscle fibers) could possibly diminish the chances of hypertensive individuals developing diabetes. An ACE inhibitor or an ARB may also correct some of the angiotensin II–induced insulin-signaling pathway abnormalities that contribute to insulin resistance in hypertensive persons.

Up to 75% of diabetic CV and renal complications can be attributed to hypertension, especially systolic hypertension (**Figure 4.3**). High BP also contributes strikingly to the development and the progression of diabetic retinopathy, which, as previously noted, is the leading cause of newly developed blindness in the United States and other industrialized nations. Isolated systolic hypertension (ISH) is common in diabetics, and supine hypertension with orthostatic hypotension is not uncommon in diabetic persons with autonomic neuropathy.

In summary, insulin resistance or impaired insulin-mediated glucose utilization is an integral component of the cardiometabolic syndrome, which often progresses to type 2 diabetes and CVD events. Hyperinsulinemia, an important component of the cardiometabolic syndrome, may contribute to the development of hyperten-

FIGURE 4.2 — Pathogenesis of Hypertension in the Insulin-Resistant State

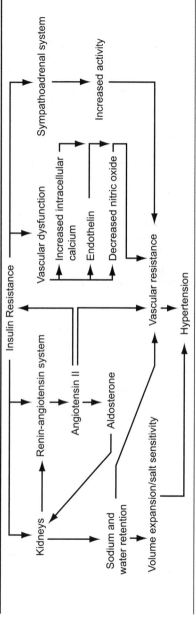

Insulin resistance involves the interaction of abnormalities of the RAAS, vascular dysfunction, the sympathetic nervous system, sodium sensitivity, and hypertension. These mechanisms are closely related in the genesis of cardiovascular events.

FIGURE 4.3 — Relationship of Elevated Systolic Blood Pressure and Complications of Diabetes

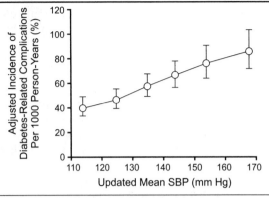

As SBP rises, diabetic CV complications increase.

Adler AI, et al. *BMJ*. 2000;321:412-419.

sion, another important component of this syndrome. Hyperinsulinemia may directly contribute to elevated BP by enhancing sympathetic nervous system activity and promoting renal sodium retention. Insulin may also indirectly increase BP by decreasing the signaling processes that are important for vascular relaxation. Further, an overexpression of the tissue renin-angiotensin system (RAS) appears to contribute to impaired insulin utilization in skeletal muscle and fat tissue, as well as diminished vasorelaxation. Therapeutic strategies that may improve insulin sensitivity, including those that interrupt the renin-angiotensin-aldosterone system (RAAS), may impede the progression of impaired insulin sensitivity to that of clinical diabetes, although this has not been proven. It has been demonstrated, however, that the use of these agents results in fewer cases of NOD than the use of some other antihypertensive agents. While some investigators do not believe that it is important to diagnose people who have the above cluster of risk factors as a "syndrome" and that treatment of a diabetic hypertensive, for example, will not differ if a patient also has visceral obesity or high triglyceride/low HDL levels, many others believe that making the diagnosis will lead to a more aggressive treatment approach.

Persons displaying impaired carbohydrate tolerance/insulin resistance as a part of the cardiometabolic syndrome and persons with diabetes often do not have a normal circadian rhythm of BP and heart rate (**Table 4.3**). These persons do not display the normal "dipping" of BP that occurs during sleep and are thus termed "nondippers" (<10-15 mm Hg decrease in SBP) (**Figure 4.4**). There are other disorders associated with nondipping, such as heart failure, autonomic neuropathy, left ventricular hypertrophy (LVH), and sleep disturbances. Nondipping in diabetics may be explained by autonomic neuropathy and impaired baroreflex function. Other factors that may play a role include intravascular volume expansion, cardiac diastolic dysfunction, and enhanced sympathetic/reduced parasympathetic and/or increased RAS activity. One caveat of nondipping is that the daytime determination of BP in such patients may represent an underestimation of the pressure load over 24 hours. Elevated nighttime BP has been found to correlate better with microalbuminuria and LVH than casual clinic BPs. The nondipping phenomenon provides additional support for more rigorous BP control in diabetics if only daytime BP readings are available.

TABLE 4.3 — Hemodynamic Characteristics of Hypertension in Diabetes

- Increased peripheral vascular resistance
- Enhanced vasoconstrictor responses to vasoagonists
- Decreased vasorelaxation responses, particularly to stimulators of nitric oxide
- Expanded plasma volume
- Supine hypertension with orthostatic hypotension
- Increased incidence of isolated systolic hypertension
- Nondipping of blood pressure at night
- Diminished baroreceptor sensitivity
- Labile hypertension

FIGURE 4.4 — 24-Hour Systolic Blood Pressure Measurements

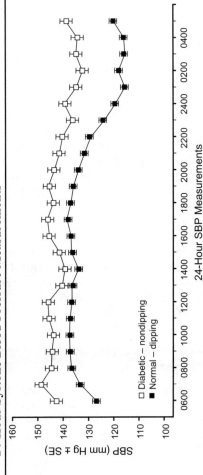

Diabetic patients frequently do not exhibit the normal decrease of about 10% in BP during sleep. This "nondipping" status and increased BP during the night may contribute to more vascular injury.

Diabetic Nephropathy

Hypertension often antedates and appears to contribute to the development of diabetic renal disease. Diabetic nephropathy, which is present after approximately 15 years of diabetes in one third of people with type 1 diabetes and in 20% of those with type 2 diabetes, is an important contributing factor for the development of hypertension in the diabetic individual. Elevated BP associated with diabetic nephropathy is usually characterized by salt and fluid retention and increased peripheral vascular resistance.

Increased vascular resistance and enhanced vasoconstricting responses to vasoagonists, such as angiotensin II, endothelin, and norepinephrine, are found early in the development of hypertension in both type 1 and type 2 diabetes. These enhanced vascular reactivity responses may reflect endothelial dysfunction (ie, decreased availability of a powerful vasodilator, nitric oxide [NO]) and small expansions in intravascular volume. Diabetic patients also display reduced baroreceptor sensitivity even prior to overt neuropathy. This reduced baroreflex sensitivity likely contributes to labile hypertension, orthostatic hypotension, and nondipping (**Table 4.3**). Also, it is becoming increasingly clear that obesity and other components of the cardiometabolic syndrome have adverse effects on the kidney, contributing to the CKD epidemic that is emerging in this country.

Dyslipidemia and Diabetes

For any lipoprotein level, diabetics have more CHD than do nondiabetics. The elevation of triglycerides and the increase in oxidation of lipoproteins that exist in the presence of hyperglycemia are cytotoxic to vascular endothelial cells and help to accelerate atherogenesis. The "diabetogenic" lipid profile consists of elevated triglycerides, reduced HDL, and very atherogenic oxidized, glycated, small, dense LDL particles.

Because of the atherogenic lipid profile and the fact, as noted previously, that diabetics are at high risk for CVD, it is generally recommended that all diabetic persons undergo a secondary prevention approach, with LDL being lowered to <100 mg/dL, HDL increased to >45 mg/dL, and triglycerides decreased to <200 mg/dL if at all possible—just as if they already had experienced a vascular event. Data suggest that in these high-risk patients, an LDL target of <70 mg/dL leads to a better outcome than a target level of <100 mg/dL.

Endothelial Dysfunction

Recognition of the importance of the vascular endothelium in maintaining vascular health has evolved over the past decade. NO, a potent vasodilator derived from vascular endothelial and smooth muscle cells, is an important modulator of local vascular tone, platelet aggregation and adhesion, and thrombus formation. Abnormal vascular NO metabolism has been observed in diabetes, hypertension, dyslipidemia, unstable angina, and CHF. These abnormalities may occur due to decreased production and/or increased destruction of NO produced by the vasculature. Superoxide anions generated by oxidative stress as a result of normal metabolism interact with NO, reducing its functional properties and promoting the formation of substances that cause cellular damage. Oxidative stress is a result of the excess generation of toxic oxygen free radicals which may occur with smoking or excessive activity of the RAAS. Inhibition of the ACE and decreased conversion of angiotensin I to angiotensin II have been shown to improve endothelial function in patients with coronary artery disease and associated CVD risks.

Hyperglycemia, hypertension, and dyslipidemia act cumulatively to cause endothelial dysfunction (**Table 4.4**). Hyperglycemia causes enhanced destruction of NO. Hyperglycemia also enhances other processes of importance in the progression of atherogenesis; enzymes involved in collagen synthesis increase when hyperglycemia is present with a tendency for increased thrombus formation.

TABLE 4.4 — Some of the Alterations in Vascular Endothelium Associated With Diabetes and Hypertension

- Increased synthesis and plasma level of endothelin-1 (a vasoconstrictive substance)
- Decreased prostacyclin release (a vasodilator substance)
- Increased destruction of endothelium-derived relaxing factor (NO) and decreased responsiveness to NO
- Impaired fibrinolytic activity
- Increased endothelial cell procoagulant activity
- Increased levels of advanced glycosylated end products
- Increased superoxide anion generation

Coagulation Abnormalities in Diabetes and Hypertension

Persons with diabetes and hypertension are prone to thrombosis because of a complex interplay among enhanced coagulation factors and diminished fibrinolytic activities, enhanced platelet aggregation, and endothelial dysfunction. A procoagulant state in diabetes is mediated, in part, by higher than normal levels of several coagulation factors (**Table 4.5**).

Plasma levels of lipoprotein (a) (Lp[a]) and PAI-1 have been reported to be elevated in diabetic patients, particularly those with poor glycemic control. By inhibiting fibrinolysis, Lp(a) and PAI-1 may delay thrombolysis and thus contribute to atherosclerotic plaque progression.

Inhibition of clot formation is modulated by specific factors that inhibit one or more of the clotting factors (antithrombin III, proteins C and S) and by the fibrino-

TABLE 4.5 — Coagulation and Fibrinolytic Abnormalities in Diabetes and Hypertension

- Elevated levels of factors VII and VIII
- Increased fibrinogen and plasminogen activator inhibitor-1 levels
- Elevated lipoprotein (a) levels
- Elevated thrombin-antithrombin complexes
- Decreased antithrombin III, protein C and S levels
- Decreased plasminogen activators and fibrinolytic activity

lytic system. In diabetic patients, fibrinolytic activity is decreased. Decreased levels of fibrinolytic factors have been found to be inversely related to glycemia as measured by glycosylated hemoglobin (HbA_{1C}) levels. Coagulation abnormalities contribute to the marked propensity for hypercoagulability in the diabetic hypertensive individual.

Platelet Abnormalities in Diabetes

4

Platelet aggregation and adhesion are characteristically enhanced in diabetes (**Table 4.6**). The cause of this enhanced platelet reactivity is complex and incompletely understood. Whether the cause relates to increases in intracellular calcium, release of certain growth factors, serotonin, or increased destruction of NO, the end result is a tendency for diabetic patients to experience more clotting disorders than nondiabetics.

TABLE 4.6 — Platelet Function Abnormalities in Diabetes and Hypertension

- Increase occurs in:
  - Platelet adhesiveness and aggregation
  - Platelet generation of vasoconstrictor prostanoids
- Decrease occurs in:
  - Platelet survival
  - Platelet generation of prostacyclin and other vasodilator prostanoids
  - Platelet production of nitric oxide
- Alteration occurs in platelet divalent cation homeostasis (decreased Mg^{2+} and increased Ca^{2+})

Microalbuminuria and CVD in Diabetes and Hypertension

There is considerable evidence that the presence of hypertension in type 1 diabetes is a consequence rather than a cause of renal disease. For example, with low levels of microalbuminuria, BP usually remains at normal levels, a finding that suggests the nephropathy precedes the rise in BP. Regardless of whether hypertension in type 1 diabetes is an etiologic factor of nephropathy or a complication of the disease, a genetic predisposition to hypertension is important in the development of nephropathy in approximately 30% of type 1 diabetics who develop this complication. It is also clear that nephropathy and hypertension accelerate each other in a logarithmic fashion.

The normal rate of protein excretion in healthy adults is <150 mg/day. Less than 30 mg of this is albumin, which has a molecular weight just large enough to keep it from passing through the normal, intact glomerulus. The remaining urine protein is comprised of different proteins and glucoproteins from tubular epithelial cells. Albumin, however, accounts for most of the protein in the urine in proteinuria due to glomerular injury, the major pathologic form of proteinuria in diabetic patients. The glomerular disease seen with diabetes is most commonly diffuse glomerulosclerosis.

The glomerular damage associated with diabetes occurs as a result of several mechanisms. One mechanism is that of glomerular capillary hypertension that leads to increased filtration and an interstitial inflammatory reaction. Glomerular capillary hypertension also increases mechanical stretch and pressure in residual glomeruli, which results in localized production of additional angiotensin II, and other factors that contribute to collagen synthesis.

Early proteinuria (microalbuminuria) is associated with endothelial cell dysfunction, enhanced oxidative stress, increased inflammation, impaired fibrinolysis, elevated SBP, nondipping, smoking, a high-salt diet, and a diabetic dyslipidemia.

Microalbuminuria, defined as 30 to 300 mg/day urinary protein, is an independent risk factor for development of CVD and a predictor of CV mortality in the diabetic population (**Figure 4.5**). It has been correlated with insulin resistance, atherogenic dyslipidemia, central obesity, and the absence of a nocturnal drop in both SBP and diastolic blood pressure (DBP), and it is a part of the metabolic CV syndrome associated with hypertension (Syndrome X) (**Table 4.7**). There is a strong association between microalbuminuria and insulin resistance. Microalbuminuria may precede and even predict the

FIGURE 4.5 — Microalbuminuria and Ischemic Heart Disease Risk

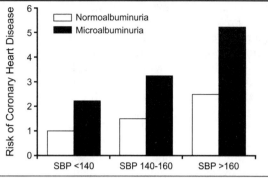

The presence of microalbuminuria (24-hour excretion of between 30 and 300 mg/d urinary protein) is associated with an increased risk of CHD at all levels of SBP. ($n=2085$; 10-year follow-up).

Borch-Johnsen K, et al. *Arterioscler Thromb Vasc Biol.* 1999;19:1992.

TABLE 4.7 — Cardiovascular Risk Factors That Tend to Cluster With Microalbuminuria

- Systolic hypertension >135 mm Hg
- Insulin resistance
- Low HDL cholesterol levels
- High triglyceride levels
- Central obesity
- Absent nocturnal drop in BP
- Salt sensitivity
- Male gender
- Increased CV oxidative stress
- Impaired endothelial function
- Abnormal coagulation/fibrinolytic profiles

onset of type 2 diabetes. It is related to endothelial dysfunction and increased oxidative stress. Therefore, it is not surprising that diabetic glomerulosis parallels diabetic vascular atherosclerosis and that microalbuminuria is an important predictor of CHD and stroke in persons with the cardiometabolic syndrome and in diabetic persons.

Numerous studies have linked microalbuminuria to other CVD risk factors. These observations collectively indicate that microalbuminuria clusters with most of the other CVD risk factors and that it reflects generalized CV/renal endothelial dysfunction and enhanced oxidative stress. Proteinuria appears to be a relatively strong surrogate marker for endothelial dysfunction and accelerated atherosclerosis. Patients with proteinuria have greater left ventricular mass, greater carotid medial thickening, and endothelial dysfunction. They have a greater propensity for MI and stroke and greater mortality with these events.

In summary, CVD is a major cause of morbidity and mortality in individuals with diabetes. Many factors, including hypertension, contribute to the high prevalence of CVD in this population. Hypertension occurs approximately twice as frequently in patients with diabetes compared with patients without diabetes. In addition, up to 75% of CVD in patients with diabetes may be attributed to hypertension, leading to recommendations for more aggressive BP control (ie, <130/80-85 mm Hg) in persons with coexistent diabetes and hypertension. Increasing obesity further contributes to both diabetes and hypertension and significantly increases CVD morbidity and mortality.

Both hygienic measures (weight loss and aerobic exercise) as well as treatment strategies that include aspirin, statins, insulin sensitizers, and antihypertensive agents that reduce RAAS activity have been shown to reduce inflammation, coagulation abnormalities, endothelial function, proteinuria, and in some cases, CVD and renal disease progression. Additional therapeutic agents are currently being developed to specifically improve insulin sensitivity and other CVD risk factors.

Relationships Between Microproteinuria, Glucose Metabolism, and Diabetes

Glucose metabolism, as measured by the insulin-clamp technique, has been observed to be impaired in normotensive type 2 diabetic persons with microalbuminuria compared with normotensive normoalbuminuric persons; the defect in insulin sensitivity was shown to correlate with urinary albumin excretion. The insulin-clamp technique measures the amount of insulin required to maintain a near optimal level of serum glucose. Insulin resistance is measured by the amount of insulin required. Several laboratories also have found that insulin sensitivity was not diminished in healthy type 2 diabetic subjects unless microalbuminuria or hypertension or both were also present. These investigations thus add to data that establish an important link between insulin resistance and the development of microalbuminuria in persons with type 2 diabetes.

The link between insulin resistance and microalbuminuria extends to persons without clinical evidence of diabetes. A publication described a group of nondiabetic, normotensive, first-degree relatives of patients with type 2 DM who were insulin resistant and also had microalbuminuria. Persons with microalbuminuria who had not developed clinical diabetes after 3.5 years still manifested multiple CVD risk factors, including hypertension, dyslipidemia (characterized by low HDL and elevated triglycerides), and high plasma levels of insulin, all components of the insulin-resistant syndrome associated with hypertension.

Thus diabetes and hypertension are closely related to several important metabolic disorders in addition to renal factors that may be noted clinically even before a diagnosis of diabetes is made. This should heighten the awareness of physicians to intervene as early as possible in as many areas as possible when patients present with elements of the diabetes-hypertension-metabolic syndrome—lower BP, attempt to correct lipid abnormalities, employ methods to prevent clotting, and promote weight loss and exercise to decrease insulin resistance and possibly improve endothelial cell dysfunction.

The Kidney: Microalbuminuria and Progression of Renal Disease

Epidemiologic studies indicate that elevated BP, especially SBP, is associated with progression of diabetic nephropathy to ESRD. To date, it appears that the two most important factors in preventing ESRD in diabetic patients are:

- Glucose and BP control prior to the development of diabetic nephropathy
- Rigorous BP control if evidence of nephropathy is present.

Once evidence of kidney involvement is present (>30 mg/day proteinuria), reduction of BP, especially SBP, is by far the most important intervention that can be undertaken to prevent progression of diabetic renal disease. A review of clinical studies on renal disease progression in diabetic patients indicated that BP reductions to levels of <130/80-85 mm Hg appear to provide protection against progression of diabetic nephropathy. There is evidence that it is important to include an ACE inhibitor or an ARB as a component of antihypertensive therapy to maximize renal protection. In most cases, the addition of a diuretic or other medication will be necessary to lower BP to goal levels.

Microalbuminuria (30-300 mg/day) is not usually detectable on a standard dipstick test. A spot morning urine measurement of albumin and creatinine is probably the most effective ascertainment of microproteinuria. A value >0.03 indicates that albuminuria is present. The amount of creatinine is determined to indicate the percentage of the 24-hour urine excreted in the overnight specimen. Normally, the total 24-hour creatinine output is about 1.2 to 1.4 g. In diabetic patients treated with antihypertensive agents, a spot morning urine albumin/creatinine should be checked at 6 months after initiating or intensifying therapy, and then generally at yearly intervals (most laboratories will report this ratio on a routine specimen).

Since a progressive increase in albuminuria is a risk factor for CVD as well as progressive nephropathy, treatment strategies that have been shown to affect the progression of microalbuminuria and renal disease include both blood glucose and BP control. Data that were reported from a multicenter Veterans Administration trial indicated that intensive glycemic control over a 2-year period reduced the progression to greater proteinuria but did not lessen the deterioration in creatinine clearance.

A number of clinical trials in diabetic patients have demonstrated that lowering BP will reduce proteinuria. A meta-analysis of clinical trials where ACE inhibitors were given (usually with other medications which most often included a thiazide diuretic) in diabetic patients with microalbuminuria found that progression from micro-albuminuria to macroalbuminuria was reduced by 79%. Regression to albumin-free urine occurred more than twice as often with an ACE inhibitor–based treatment strategy than with a regimen that did not include an ACE inhibitor. Treatment effect was unaltered by glycemic control, BP, gender, or age and seemed to be greater in patients with diabetes of longer duration.

Three trials have also established that treatment regimens that include an ARB will decrease renal disease progression when compared with a program that does not include an ARB or ACE inhibitor (see *Chapter 6* for details of these studies—Reduction of Endpoints in Noninsulin Dependent Diabetes Mellitus With an Angiotensin II Antagonist, Losartan [RENAAL], Irbesartan Diabetic Nephropathy Trial [IDNT], and Irbesartan Microalbuminuria Type 2 Diabetes Mellitus in Hypertension Patients Trial [IRMA 2]).

Recent data from the Ongoing Telmisartan Alone or in Combination With Ramipril Global Endpoint Trial (ONTARGET) suggest that while BP may be decreased to a somewhat greater degree with an ARB plus an ACE inhibitor compared with an ACE inhibitor alone, the combination of these two classes of drugs may actually have an adverse effect on renal function. In this trial, about 37% of patients were diabetics; no difference in outcome between these patients and nondiabetics was noted.

Finally, there are emerging data suggesting that lipid treatment, particularly with statins, can reduce the progression of proteinuria and CKD in persons with the metabolic syndrome and diabetes.

It should be reemphasized that in all of these trials, other medications (most often a diuretic) were required to decrease BP toward a goal level. Thus the treated hypertensive patient in whom microalbuminuria persists should have their BP treatment intensified. This most often requires the use of several antihypertensive agents, which should include a diuretic. Concomitant therapies with lipid-lowering agents and aspirin should also be undertaken (**Figure 4.6**). **Table 4.8** summarizes the significance of microproteinuria and how it is measured.

FIGURE 4.6 — Association of Microalbuminuria and Cardiovascular Morbidity and Mortality in Type 2 Diabetes

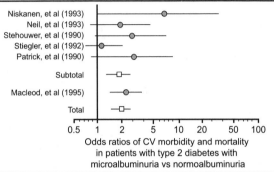

Odds ratios of CV morbidity and mortality in patients with type 2 diabetes with microalbuminuria vs normoalbuminuria

Microalbuminuria is a strong predictor of all-cause mortality and CV morbidity and mortality in type 2 diabetes. A meta-analysis of prospective trials of patients with type 2 diabetes found an overall OR of 3.1 for total mortality and 1.8 for CV morbidity and mortality in patients with microproteinuria. Although the mechanism underlying the association between microalbuminuria and mortality is not clear, the presence of microalbuminuria may reflect a generalized defect in vascular permeability leading to atherogenesis. Hypertension is a major risk factor for the development of microalbuminuria.

Dinneen SF, Gerstein HC. *Arch Intern Med*. 1997;157:1413-1418.

TABLE 4.8 — Microalbuminuria

What is it?

Excretion of small amounts (30-300 mg/d) of protein in the urine

How it is determined?

Spot morning urine sample for protein (creatinine levels in the urine to determine the percentage of 24-h urine volume excreted). Use albumin-to-creatinine ratio; >0.03 indicates proteinuria

What testing methods are available?

Micral II dipstick ($4 to $7/strip) and spot urine for albumin-to-creatinine ratio ($12 to $14/sample)

What does it mean?

Is suggestive of vascular injury not just in the kidney but in blood vessels elsewhere (correlates with CV risk)

What should be done about it?

Glycemic control; control of BP to levels <130-135/80-85 mm Hg

Is specific therapy indicated?

The use of an ACE inhibitor or an ARB usually with a diuretic; probably represents the most appropriate therapy to lower BP and reduce proteinuria

SUGGESTED READING

DREAM Trial Investigators; Bosch J, Yusuf S, Gerstein HC, et al. Effect of ramipril on the incidence of diabetes. *N Engl J Med.* 2006;355:1551-1562.

Chen J, Muntner P, Hamm LL, et al. The metabolic syndrome and chronic kidney disease in U.S. adults. *Ann Intern Med.* 2004;140:167-174.

Jee SH, Boulware LE, Guallar E, Suh I, Appel LJ, Miller ER 3rd. Direct, progressive association of cardiovascular risk factors with incident proteinuria: results from the Korea Medical Insurance Corporation (KMIC) study. *Arch Intern Med.* 2005;165:2299-2304.

McFarlane SI, Castro J, Kaur J, et al. Control of blood pressure and other cardiovascular risk factors at different pratice settings: outcomes of care provided to diabetic women compared to men. *J Clin Hyperten.* 2005;3:235-241.

Moser M, Falkner B, Weber MA, Keilson LM. The metabolic syndrome—what is it and how should it be managed? *J Clin Hyper.* 2006;8:44-49.

ONTARGET Investigators, Yusuf S, Teo KK, Pogue J, et al. Telmisartan, ramipril, or both in patients at high risk for vascular events. *N Engl J Med.* 2008;358:1547-1459.

Sowers JR. Metabolic risk factors and renal disease. *Kidney Int.* 2007;71:719-720.

5

The Renin-Angiotensin-Aldosterone System in Diabetes

Insulin resistance plays an important role in promoting hypertension in patients with the cardiometabolic syndrome. The RAAS also appears to play an important role in the development of hypertension in diabetic patients. It exerts its hypertensive action via stimulation of salt and water retention, increasing vascular tone and interference with the vasorelaxing action of insulin. Effects of the RAAS are not limited to regulation of vascular tone but are more pleiotropic. This system is necessary to sustain CV function, particularly with relation to maintaining plasma volume. Chronic overactivity, however, leads to maladaptive tissue responses such as a permanent increase of vascular resistance, myocardial fibrosis and hypertrophy, endothelial dysfunction, decreased stability of atherosclerotic plaques, and reduced fibrinolysis/increased coagulation.

■ The RAAS in Diabetes

The relationship between the RAAS and insulin signaling is complex and involves several intracellular mechanisms and signaling pathways. Normally, insulin binds to its receptor on the surface of insulin-sensitive cells and triggers a series of reactions in insulin receptor substances that aid in glucose transport. Activation of the angiotensin II (AT_1) receptor decreases insulin's ability to stimulate glucose transport; this leads to insulin resistance (more insulin is required to maintain a stable serum glucose level). ACE inhibitor therapy improves insulin sensitivity, in part, by overcoming some of these effects of angiotensin II on insulin-stimulated glucose transport in skeletal muscle tissue. ARBs are also effective in reducing the activity of angiotensin II in peripheral tissues.

Cardiomyopathy, one of the complications of diabetes, may be linked to activation of the local RAAS in the heart. Angiotensinogen, renin, and AT_1 receptor concentrations are increased in the heart of diabetic animals. This increased RAAS expression in the heart leads to increased fibrosis, altered NO metabolism, reduced sodium pump and potassium channel expression/activity, and delayed diastolic relaxation that characterizes diabetic cardiomyopathy. These observations may also explain why ACE inhibitor and aldosterone antagonists have proven beneficial in diabetic patients with CVD. ACE inhibitors and ARBs appear to exert beneficial effects on both left ventricular diastolic and systolic function. Improved cardiac function also appears to influence the rate of albumin excretion in patients with overt or preclinical diabetic nephropathy.

Strategies for Inhibition of the RAAS

As shown in **Figure 5**.1, there are several pharmacologic approaches for inhibition of the RAAS, which include inhibition of the ACE with ACE inhibitors, blockade of the AT_1 receptors with ARBs, and direct inhibition of renin.

ACE is a key enzyme in the activation of the RAAS, which helps to convert angiotensin I (an inactive substance) to angiotensin II. In addition, it inactivates vasodilatory kinins (such as bradykinin) (**Figure 5**.1). Angiotensin II and aldosterone are major hormones that exert their actions to maintain fluid volume and promote increased vasomotor tone. They are produced by the heart, kidney, and the vasculature where they have local actions. ACE inhibitors block the generation of angiotensin II and increase the availability of vasodilating substances such as bradykinin. There are several angiotensin II receptors: AT_1 is the major receptor controlling vasomotor tone and is the receptor inhibited by the ARBs.

Renin, which is secreted by the kidney in response to decreases in blood volume and renal perfusion, cleaves angiotensinogen to angiotensin I. Thus, inhibition of renin activity can lead, ultimately, to decreased production of angiotensin II. (See *Chapter 7* for a discussion of the direct renin inhibitor, aliskiren.)

FIGURE 5.1—Site of Action of ACE Inhibitors, Angiotensin II Receptor Blockers, and Renin Inhibitors

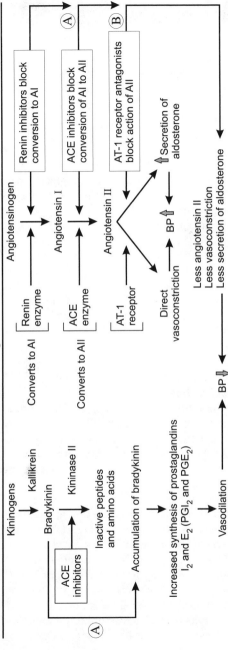

(A) Mode of action of direct renin inhibitors: block cleavage of angiotensinogen to angiotensin I. (B) Mode of action of ACE inhibitors: block conversion of AI (an inactive substance) to AII (a vasoconstrictor). This action (1) decreases the generation of AII, and also by blocking the activity of kininase II, (2) decreases the breakdown of bradykinin; this vasodilator substance increases and BP is lowered. (C) Mode of action of AII receptor blockers (AT-1): block effects of AII peripherally; aldosterone secretion is not increased and vasoconstriction is prevented; no effect on bradykinin system; does not prevent production of AII.

73

■ **Nephropathy**

ACE inhibitors, when given as part of a treatment regimen, protect against deterioration of renal function in diabetic nephropathy; their use may produce benefits in addition to BP control. In the Heart Outcomes Prevention Evaluation and Microalbuminuria, Cardiovascular, and Renal Outcomes (MICRO-HOPE) study, a dose of ramipril (an ACE inhibitor) 10 mg per day in addition to other medications lowered the risk of overt nephropathy by 24% in a group of high-risk patients compared with subjects who did not receive ACE inhibitor therapy as part of a treatment regimen. These results suggest that ACE inhibitor therapy may be particularly beneficial in diabetic patients who have cardiac and renal disease. Data also suggest that ARBs have a similar action. As noted, the use of a β-blocker/diuretic treatment program will also reduce proteinuria and at least in one trial (UKPDS), these therapies were as effective in reducing morbidity/mortality as an ACE inhibitor–based program in diabetic patients whose blood pressure was lowered more than another group (see *Chapter 6*).

■ **Insulin Resistance and the Development of New-Onset Diabetes**

The Captopril Prevention Project (CAPPP) was a randomized study which reported that the group of hypertensive patients treated with captopril, an ACE inhibitor, had a significantly lower rate of development of NOD when compared with the group of patients receiving conventional therapy.

In addition, during the 5-year follow-up period of the HOPE trial, there was a 34% reduction in the development of NOD in patients receiving the ACE inhibitor compared with the non–ACE inhibitor-treated group. *In all of the trials in hypertensive diabetes, multiple medications were usually necessary to lower BP to goal levels.* In most of the trials, a large percentage of patients were receiving a diuretic in addition to the study drugs.

Studies have shown that ACE inhibitors increase insulin sensitivity and improve glycemic control in patients with clinical DM. The results of the MICRO-HOPE trial showed that diabetic patients taking ramipril (plus other medications) achieved better-control of their diabetes than patients taking medications that did not include an ACE inhibitor. Compared with baseline, mean absolute HbA_{1C} values were 1.5% higher than the upper limit of normal in the ramipril group and 3.4% higher in the other group at 1 year. At 2 years, HbA_{1C} decreased by 0.1% in participants taking ramipril and rose by 2.2% in participants taking other medications that did not include an ACE inhibitor. Similar results were reported by the EURODIAB Controlled Trial of Lisinopril in Insulin-Dependent Diabetes Mellitus (EUCLID) study, which showed that HbA_{1C} was significantly lower in a lisinopril (ACE inhibitor)–treated group than in a group of patients on other medications. An increased incidence of hypoglycemia has been reported in diabetic patients receiving a combination of an ACE inhibitor and oral hypoglycemic agents or insulin. This suggests that ACE inhibitor therapy increases insulin sensitivity in people with insulin resistance, including patients with hypertension.

The mechanism by which ACE inhibitors improve insulin sensitivity in patients with diabetes, hypertension, and the metabolic CV syndrome is complex and not completely understood. One effect involves improvement in blood flow to insulin-resistant muscles.

It has been observed that ACE inhibitors facilitate blood flow through the microcirculation in skeletal muscles. This effect is bradykinin-dependent. As noted in **Figure 5.1**, ACE inhibitor therapy prolongs the action of bradykinin by blocking its breakdown and facilitating its action on receptors. Bradykinin not only causes vasodilation but also independently increases the basal and insulin-stimulated rate of glucose uptake in skeletal muscle in insulin-resistant states. Thus ACE inhibitors may mediate improvements in insulin activity, at least in part, through bradykinin-mediated mechanisms. This specific action on bradykinin is not noted with the use of an ARB, which does not interfere with its degradation.

A review of data on the occurrence of NOD in hypertensive patients treated with antihypertensive medications indicates the following:

- Hypertensives develop diabetes more frequently than normotensive individuals.
- The use of diuretics compared with placebo may increase NOD by approximately 0.6% to about 1.5% (**Table 5.1**).
- β-Blockers increase NOD by about 7.3/1000 patient years compared with no therapy.
- Comparative clinical trials with different medications where patient populations vary considerably indicate that NOD occurs approximately 2% to 3% less frequently with agents that block the RAAS system (eg, ACE inhibitors and ARBs) when compared with treatments that did not include these agents (**Table 5.2** and **Table 5.3**).

These data add to the recommendation that in obese subjects or patients with manifestations of the metabolic syndrome, an RAAS inhibitor should be part of the treatment program.

■ Vascular Health in the Diabetic Patient With Hypertension

To reemphasize, ACE inhibitors reduce oxidation of LDL, decrease fibrinogen levels, reduce oxidative stress, and normalize endothelial NO function, both by increased production and by decreased destruction of NO. Improvement of insulin-mediated vascular relaxation is noted. ACE inhibition also decreases secretion of endothelin-1, which is a potent vasoconstrictor and a mitogenic factor for vascular smooth muscle cells and fibroblasts via bradykinin, an NO-dependent mechanism. ACE inhibitors may also diminish expression of adhesion molecules by the endothelium and decrease cytokine-induced inflammation, both of which are important in the atherogenic process that is enhanced in diabetic vasculature.

Several trials have indicated that in patients with diabetes and hypertension, ACE inhibitors appear to be more effective than other treatment modalities in terms of reduction of risk of CVD events. In the HOPE study in very high-risk patients who were on multiple medications, the addition of an ACE inhibitor (ramipril) lowered

TABLE 5.1 — Effects of Moderate- and High-Dose Diuretic Therapy on Glucose Metabolism in Placebo-Controlled Trials

Study	Duration (y)	Serum Glucose (mg/dL)	Hyperglycemia or Diabetes
Oslo	5	No difference—diuretics; placebo	No specific data available
EWPHE	3	Increase 6.6—diuretics; placebo	Excess of 6/1000 patient years
MRC	3	No specific data available	Excess of 6/1000 patient years
HAPPHY	4	No specific data available	Excess of 6/1000 patient years
HDFP	5	No specific data available	1.6% (57/3563)
SHEP	3	Difference of 4 mg/dL—drug vs placebo in diabetics	1 of 483
		Difference of 3 mg/dL in nondiabetics	No significant difference in number of new cases of diabetes in treatment group compared with placebo group
ALLHAT	At 4+	Increase of 3 mg/dL (ACE inhibitor ↓ 1 mg/dL)	3.5% more new-onset diabetes with diuretics compared with ACE inhibitors[a]
VA	2	Increase of 1.7—diuretics; placebo	No specific data available
TOMHS	1	Decrease of 0.9—diuretics; decrease of 3.2—placebo	No specific data available

[a] Fasting glucose >126 mg/dL.

Modified and updated from: *Cleve Clin J Med.* 1993;60:27-37.

5

TABLE 5.2 — New-Onset Diabetes in the Prospective, Comparative, Randomized Hypertension Treatment Trials (3 to 8 Years' Follow-Up)[a]

Trial (N)	Duration (y)	Therapy	New-Onset Diabetes (%)	Absolute Difference (%)
ALLHAT (21,294)	5+	Diuretic	11.6	—
		ACE inhibitor	8.1	3.5
		CCB	9.8	1.8
ANBP-2 (5626)	4+	Diuretic	6.56	
		ACE inhibitor	4.54	2.02
CAPPP (10,985)	6+	β-Blocker and diuretic	7.3	
		ACE inhibitor	6.5	0.8
CHARM (5439)	3+	Other therapy (usual care)	7.4	
		ARB	6.0	1.4
HOPE (5720)	5	Other therapy (usual care)	5.4	
		ACE inhibitor	3.6	1.8
INSIGHT (5019)	4+	Diuretic	7.0	
		CCB	5.4	1.6
INVEST (16,176)	5+	β-Blocker and diuretic	8.2	
		CCB/ACE inhibitor	7.0	1.2
LIFE (7998)	5	β-Blocker	8.0	
		ARB	6.0	2.0

78

SCOPE (4342)	5	Other therapy (usual care)	5.3	1.0
		ARB	4.3	
STOP-2 (5895)	6+	UC	4.9	—
		CCB	4.8	0.01
		ACE inhibitor	4.7	0.02
VALUE (15,245)	4+	ARB	13.1	3.3
		CCB	16.4	

[a] Multiple medications used in all trials in an effort to achieve goal BP levels; >100,000 patients.

TABLE 5.3 — Incidence of New-Onset Diabetes With Different Antihypertensive Medications in the 3- to 8-Year Hypertension Treatment Trials

Trial	Therapy	Duration (y)	New-Onset Diabetes (%)		Absolute Difference (%)
ACE-I Compared With Usual Care (D/β-Bl)			*ACE-I*	*UC or D/β-Bl*	
CAPPP	ACE-I/β-Bl/D	6.1	6.5	7.5	1.0
STOP-2	ACE-I/β-Bl/D	6+	4.7	4.9	0.2
ANBP-2	ACE-I/D	4+	4.5	6.6	2.1
ALLHAT	ACE-I/D	4.9	8.1	11.6	3.5
CCB Compared With Usual Care			*CCB*	*CT*	
NORDIL	CCB/β-Bl/D	4.5	4.3	4.9	0.6
ALLHAT	CCB/D	4.9	9.8	11.6	1.8
INVEST	CCB/β-Bl	4.0	6.2	7.3	1.1
INSIGHT	CCB/D	3.5	5.4	7.0	1.6
STOP-2	CCB/β-Bl/D	6+	4.8	4.9	0.1
ARB Compared With Other Therapies			*ARB*	*OT*	
VALUE	ARB/CCB	4.2	13.1	16.4	3.3
LIFE	ARB/β-Bl	4.8	6.0	8.0	2.0
SCOPE	ARB/UC	5	4.3	5.3	1.0
CHARM	ARB/OT	3+	6.0	7.4	1.4

ACE-I Compared With CCB

			ACE-I	CCB
ALLHAT	ACE-I/CCB	4.9	8.1	9.8	1.7

Key: ACE-I, angiotensin-converting enzyme inhibitor; ARB, angiotensin II receptor blocker; β-Bl, β-blocker; CCB, calcium channel blocker; CT, conventional therapy; D, diuretic; OT, other therapy; UC, usual care.

Approximate overall difference: ACE or ARB vs D/β-Bl = 2.0%; ACE vs CCB = 2.0%; CCB vs D/β-Bl = 1.5%.

Moser M. *J Clin Hyper*. 2004;6:610-613.

the risk of MI by 22%, stroke by 33%, CV mortality by 24%, and total mortality by 24%. These changes were achieved despite the fact that BP differences between the ACE-inhibitor–treated group and a control group were only 2.4 mm Hg systolic and 1.0 mm Hg diastolic. Some experts believe that a difference of even this magnitude may account for at least some of the benefit of treatment. There are some data in the HOPE trial, where the study drug was given in the evening, that nighttime BPs were considerably lower (based on a very small subset of patients who were studied with ambulatory BP monitoring) (see *Chapter 6* under section entitled *Heart Outcome Prevention Evaluation [HOPE] Study*).

As reviewed in *Chapter 6*, a meta-analysis of several randomized controlled trials (Appropriate Blood Pressure Control in Diabetes [ABCD], Fosinopril vs Amlodipine Cardiovascular Event Trial [FACET], and CAPPP) that included a total of 2,180 patients with type 2 diabetes and hypertension. These patients, who were treated with ACE inhibitors compared with another antihypertensive agent(s), showed a benefit with ACE inhibitors compared with alternative treatment in the outcomes of acute MI (63% reduction), CVD events (51% reduction), and all-cause mortality (62% reduction). The ABCD trial was terminated early after the benefits of ACE inhibition compared with calcium channel blockade was established. The FACET was originally designed to compare the effects of fosinopril with amlodipine on serum lipid levels and diabetic control in 380 patients with type 2 diabetes and hypertension. Even though there were no differences in glucose and lipid control in the two groups by the end of 3.5 years of follow-up, subjects assigned to fosinopril treatment were at significantly lower risk for the combined outcome of stroke, MI, and hospitalization for angina than subjects assigned to amlodipine treatment. It should be noted that patients treated with both fosinopril and amlodipine had the least CVD events. It should also be emphasized that the numbers of patients with defined end points were small in both the ABCD trial and FACET.

To recap another study (UKPDS) that compared outcomes of treatment with an ACE inhibitor (captopril)–

based treatment program and treatment with a β-blocker (atenolol)–based treatment program, both treatment regimens were found to be equally effective in reduction of CV events if strict BP control was maintained (ie, in patients who achieved the lowest BPs, events were reduced regardless of the treatment regimen). The absence of a difference in the rate of reduction of CV mortality between patients treated with different medications might partially be explained by the similarity of action of both medications in reducing activity of the RAAS, respectively (ie, β-blockers decrease renin production; ACE inhibitors decrease angiotensin II production). In the UKPDS study, microvascular complications of diabetes, such as nephropathy and retinopathy, were also benefited equally in the β-blocker and ACE groups.

Of interest is the fact that in a 10-year follow-up of the UKPDS, the benefits of initially reducing blood glucose and HbA_{1C} levels by intensive therapy to a greater degree than standard care persisted despite the lack of long-term differences in these parameters between the groups. Significant reductions in any diabetes-related end points, microvascular disease, and all-cause mortality were noted in the intensive-care group. However, the differences in outcome and benefit that were noted in the original study where BP was reduced by -10/-5 mmHg in the intensive-treatment group compared with the standard-care group did not persist as BP differences decreased over the 10-year follow-up. Results suggest that BP control must be ongoing for benefit to continue, while early glucose control may result in a reduction of CV events even if control is less satisfactory over time.

The use of ARBs which block the effects of angiotensin II at vascular receptor sites has also been shown to slow down progression of renal disease in long-term studies of type 2 diabetics with varying degrees of nephropathy.

Thus ACE inhibitors or agents that block the activity of the RAAS influence different aspects of vascular disease in the patient with diabetes and hypertension. These actions result in:

- Inhibiting the RAAS and improved insulin sensitivity

- Lowering of BP
- Decreasing oxidation of lipoproteins
- Improving endothelial function.

In patients with diabetes and/or IGT, ACE inhibition or angiotensin receptor blockade with an ARB improves glycemic control, reduces microalbuminuria, and improves renal function. All of the above suggest that medications that interfere with the RAAS are important in the management of diabetes and the metabolic syndrome, with a potential to reduce morbidity and mortality in this high-risk group. Clinical trials with ARBs and more limited data with aldosterone antagonists also suggest benefit in reducing renal and CV disease outcomes in patients with the comorbid conditions of diabetes and hypertension.

Chaturvedi N, Sjolie AK, Stephenson JM, et al. Effect of lisinopril on progression of retinopathy in normotensive people with type 1 diabetes. The EUCLID Study Group. EURODIAB controlled trial of lisinopril in insulin-dependent diabetes mellitus. *Lancet*. 1998;351:28-31.

Cooper SA, Whaley-Connel A, Habibi J, et al. Renin-angiotensin-aldosterone system oxidative stress in cardiovascular insulin resistance. *Am J Physiol Heart Circ Physiol*. 2007;293:H2009-H2023.

Fiordaliso F, Li B, Latini R, et al. Myocyte death in streptozotocin-induced diabetes in rats is angiotensin II-dependent. *Lab Invest*. 2000; 80:513-527.

Gradman AH, Traub D. The efficacy of aliskiren, a direct renin inhibitor, in the treatment of hypertension. *Rev Cardiovasc Med*. 2007;8(suppl 2):S22-S30.

Heart Outcomes Prevention Evaluation Study Investigators. Effect of ramipril on cardiovascular and microvascular outcomes in people with diabetes mellitus: results of the HOPE study and MICRO-HOPE substudy. Heart Outcomes Prevention Evaluation Study Investigators. *Lancet*. 2000;355:253-259.

Herings RM, de Boer A, Stricker BH, Leufkens HG, Porsius A. Hypo-glycaemia associated with use of inhibitors of angiotensin converting enzyme. *Lancet*. 1995;345:1195-1198.

Holman RR, Paul SK, Bethel MA, Matthews DR, Neil HA. 10-year follow-up of intensive glucose control in type 2 diabetes. *N Engl J Med*. 2008;359:1577-1589.

Holman RR, Paul SK, Bethel MA, Neil HA, Matthews DR. Long-term follow-up after tight control of blood pressure in type 2 diabetes. *N Engl J Med*. 2008;359:1565-1576.

Mathiesen ER, Hommel E, Hansen HP, Smidt UM, Parving HH. Randomised controlled trial of long term efficacy of captopril on preservation of kidney function in normotensive patients with in-sulin dependent diabetes and microalbuminuria. *BMJ*. 1999;319: 24-25.

McFarlane SI, Banerji M, Sowers JR. Insulin resistance and cardiovas-cular disease. *J Clin Endocrinol Metab*. 2001;86:713-718.

Moser M. Current hypertension management: separating fact from fic-tion. *Cleve Clin J Med*. 1993;60:27-37.

Moser M. Is new-onset diabetes of clinical significance in treated hy-pertensive patients? *J Clin Hyper*. 2006;8:126-132.

Muirhead N, Feagan BF, Mahon J, et al. The effects of valsartan and captopril on reducing microalbuminuria in patients with type 2

5

diabetes mellitus: a placebo-controlled trial. *Curr Therapeutic Res.* 1999;60:650-660.

O'Brien E, Barton J, Nussberger J, et al. Aliskiren reduces blood pressure and suppresses plasma renin activity in combination with a thiazide diuretic, an angiotensin-converting enzyme inhibitor, or an angiotensin receptor blocker. *Hypertension.* 2007;49:276-284.

Rachmani R, Lidar M, Brosh D, Levi Z, Ravid M. Oxidation of low-density lipoprotein in normotensive type 2 diabetic patients. Comparative effect of enalapril versus nifedipine: a randomized crossover study. *Diabetes Res Clin Pract.* 2000;48:139-145.

Sowers JR. Metabolic risk factors and renal disease. *Kidney Int.* 2007;71:719-720.

Sowers JR. Treatment of hypertension in patients with diabetes. *Arch Intern Med.* 2004;164:1850-1857.

Young M, Funder JW. Aldosterone and the heart. *Trends Endocrinol Metab.* 2000;11:224-226.

6

Hypertension Treatment Trials in Diabetic Patients

In view of unequivocal epidemiologic evidence that has been available for >20 to 30 years that the risk of CVD is greatly increased in diabetics, it would have seemed logical that greater efforts to reduce CVD risk factors in addition to correcting abnormal glucose metabolism in these patients might have been undertaken years ago. This is especially true in relation to hypertension. But without long-term clinical evidence that treating high BP in hypertensive diabetic patients was beneficial, many physicians had been reluctant to treat patients with diabetes with antihypertensive medications. In many of the early hypertension studies, diabetic patients were actually excluded from treatment for fear that some of the medications might adversely affect outcome.

Definitive evidence has now been available for 8 to 10 years that lowering BP will reduce morbidity and mortality in the diabetic patient, probably to a greater extent than controlling blood glucose levels. The evidence strongly suggests that in the young or old, lowering of elevated BP will be beneficial. Goal BP levels in a nondiabetic are presently set at <140/90 mm Hg; based on the fact that diabetics are at high risk, goal levels in these patients should be set at 130/80-85 mm Hg.

Early Clinical Trials in Diabetic Patients With Hypertension

■ **Hypertension Detection Follow-Up Program and the Systolic Hypertension in the Elderly Program**
In some earlier studies, ie, the Hypertension Detection Follow-up Program (HDFP) and Systolic Hypertension in the Elderly Program (SHEP), diabetes was not an exclusion criterion. In the HDFP trial, approximately 10% of the hypertensive participants were diabetics. The HDFP was a population-based trial to assess the

efficacy of an intensive stepped-care (SC) antihypertensive regimen compared with community referred care (RC) among persons with diastolic hypertension (>90 mm Hg) in preventing all-cause mortality. Initial therapy in the SC group was chlorthalidone 25 mg, which could be increased to 100 mg (a dose considered unnecessarily high at present but one which was in common use in the 1960s and 1970s). Add-on therapy included a β-blocker or reserpine and other medications (eg, hydralazine, a vasodilator) that might be necessary to reduce BP. In the RC group, diuretics and other agents were also used but presumably in lower doses.

The difference in BP between the SC and the RC groups at the end of a 5-year study was –12/–5 mm Hg. A large number of subjects did not achieve the goal DBP of ≤90 mm Hg. Of the >10,000 patients aged 30 to 69 randomized at baseline, 1079 were classified as diabetics. These included both insulin- and non–insulin-treated patients (type 1 and type 2). The diagnosis was based on a history of a fasting blood glucose of >140 mg/dL (7.8 mmol/L). This diagnostic criterion has been changed to a fasting glucose level of >126 mg/dL. Obviously, more patients would have been included if this newer definition had been used. At the end of 5 years in the nondiabetic group, the all-cause mortality rate was 17% lower in the SC group compared with the RC group. Overall, in diabetic patients, the death rate was similar for the SC and the RC groups (**Table 6.1**), but there were differences in outcome depending on the severity of the hypertension. A large HDFP subgroup had less severe degrees of hypertension (stage 1), defined at that time as a DBP 90-104 mm Hg (when the HDFP began, physicians paid less attention to SBP). More recently, stage 1 DBP has been defined as 90-100 mm Hg. In this group of less-severe hypertensives, 466 were diabetic. All-cause mortality was lower in the SC group of less-severe hypertensives than in the RC group for both diabetic and nondiabetic patients (20.5% and 22.2%, respectively) (**Table 6.1**) despite the fact that presently defined goal BPs were not achieved in many patients.

It is well known that the outlook for untreated hypertensive diabetic patients is considerably less favorable

TABLE 6.1 — Hypertension Detection and Follow-Up Program Results in Diabetic Subjects[a]

	Nondiabetics	Diabetics
5-Year all-cause mortality	17% lower in SC group	No difference between SC and RC groups
Patients with DBPs 90-104 mm Hg (466 patients)	22.2% lower in SC group	20.5% lower in SC group[b]

[a] 1079 patients with history of diabetes or fasting blood sugar ≥140 mg/dL.

[b] Although the relative decrease in mortality was similar in the diabetic subjects, the baseline absolute risk was greater in diabetic subjects and absolute benefits were greater in those individuals.

than for untreated nondiabetic hypertensive individuals. *At similar levels of BP, there is an increased morbidity/ mortality in untreated hypertensive diabetics compared with nondiabetics.* Thus while the relative risk of mortality was reduced equally by about 20% to 22% in diabetics and nondiabetics who received more-aggressive therapy compared with less-aggressive treatment, the absolute risk reduction was greater in the diabetic patients because of the greater baseline risk.

These findings of benefit in this subgroup of SC diabetic patients with initial DBP of 90-104 mm Hg are similar to the SHEP findings. SHEP was a study of >5000 people >60 years of age with ISH, defined at that time as SBP >160 mm Hg and DBP ≤90 mm Hg. There were 583 patients (12%) with diabetes. This included patients with a history of diabetes, patients on oral hypoglycemic agents, and patients with fasting serum glucose levels >140 mg/dL. In this study, chlorthalidone (12.5 to 25 mg/ day) was the initial drug of choice with atenolol (25 to 50 mg/day) added if necessary. The treated group consisted of 283 patients; 300 patients were given a placebo.

At the end of year 4, about one third of the treated patients were receiving both chlorthalidone and another agent, usually atenolol. In the diabetic patients, BP was lowered by −10/2 mm Hg in the treated group compared with the placebo group. At the end of the treatment period, in diabetic patients there was a significant reduction of 56% in all major CHD events. This compares with a reduction of 19% in the treated nondiabetic patients compared with those who received placebo (**Figure 6.1**). Nonfatal MI and fatal CHD events were also reduced significantly more in the treated diabetic patients than in nondiabetics compared with the placebo groups; a reduction in risk of 54% in the diabetic patients and 23% in the nondiabetics compared with subjects receiving placebo. All-cause mortality was also reduced to a greater degree (26%) in the treated diabetic patients (compared with placebo) compared with 15% in the nondiabetic treated patients (compared with placebo). Fatal and nonfatal strokes, however, appeared to be reduced more in the nondiabetic cohort (**Table 6.2**): a nonsignificant reduction of –22% from placebo in diabetics and a significant

FIGURE 6.1 — **Systolic Hypertension in the Elderly Program**: **Influence of Diabetes on Cardiovascular Event Rates**

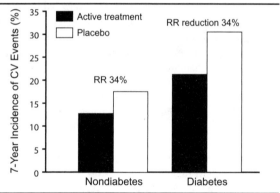

Among the 583 patients with type 2 diabetes, the 5-year major CV event rate was lower by 34% with antihypertensive therapy compared with placebo. Although an identical 34% reduction in the major CV event rate was found in nondiabetic patients, the absolute risk reduction with active treatment compared with placebo was twice as great in patients with diabetes as in those without diabetes, due to the higher absolute risk of a CV event in patients with diabetes.

Curb JD, et al. *JAMA*. 1996;276:1886-1892.

TABLE 6.2 — Cumulative 5-Year Rates (1000 Patient-Years) of Cardiovascular Events in the Systolic Hypertension in the Elderly Program

CV Event	Diabetic Group		Nondiabetic Group	
	Active Therapy	Placebo	Active Therapy	Placebo
Major CHD events	9.2	16.0	6.9	7.6
Nonfatal MI or fatal CHD	7.7	13.1	5.1	5.7
Nonfatal and fatal strokes	9.7	14.4	4.4	7.5
Major cerebrovascular disease events	21.4	31.5	13.3	10.4

Placebo-treated diabetic patients had about 2 to 3 times the risk of a CV event as placebo-treated nondiabetics.

reduction of –38% in nondiabetics compared with placebo. Reduction in all major CVD events was equal for treated diabetics and nondiabetic subjects (–34%) (**Figure 6.2**).

FIGURE 6.2 — **Morbidity and Mortality in Diabetic and Nondiabetic Subjects in the Systolic Hypertension in the Elderly Program**[a]

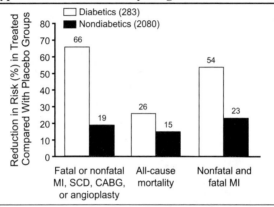

[a] Therapy: low-dose diuretic with β-blocker added if necessary; $n=4736$; subjects >60 yo.

Curb JD, et al. *JAMA*. 1996;276:1886-1892.

For all outcomes, the relative risk or reduction in events for treated diabetic patients was as favorable or more favorable than for treated nondiabetic patients. As noted earlier, since risk from hypertension is considerably higher in diabetic subjects, the absolute risk reductions with active treatment compared with placebo were consistently greater in treated diabetic patients than in treated nondiabetic patients; 101/1000 compared with 51/1000 randomized participants, respectively, had benefited from treatment at the 5-year follow-up. This reflects the higher baseline risk for diabetic hypertensive patients. For example, untreated diabetics had a cumulative 5-year rate of major CHD events of 16/100; untreated nondiabetics, a rate of only 7.6/100. Rates for nonfatal MI or fatal CHD were 13.1/100 compared with 5.7/100. *Therapy reduced the risk in diabetics in many categories to levels close to those in nondiabetic subjects*. In the nondiabetic group, lowering BP also reduced risk compared with risk in subjects with higher BP.

There was little or no evidence that adverse effects of treatment had impacted the important positive results in this randomized controlled trial. However, several adverse effects of therapy appeared to be more common in diabetics than in nondiabetics (**Table 6.3**). For example, cold or numb hands occurred in 25% of treated diabetics compared with 17% in the placebo group. Treated nondiabetics noted this symptom in 17% compared with 14% in the placebo group. It is recognized that sexual dysfunction, which is presumably secondary to vascular disease as well as autonomic nerve dysfunction, is more common in diabetic male patients. Yet in the SHEP trial, the incidence of sexual dysfunction, as well as symptoms of depression and dementia, were not statistically significantly different between treated and placebo subjects in either nondiabetics or diabetics. In general, adverse effects of therapy were not of great importance in the majority of patients.

Thus both in HDFP, which was a study of diastolic and systolic hypertension in middle-aged individuals, and in SHEP, which was a study of ISH in elderly patients

6

TABLE 6.3 — Symptoms in Active-Therapy Diabetic Subjects Compared With Placebo Subjects in the Systolic Hypertension in the Elderly Program

Symptom	Diabetics (%)	Nondiabetics (%)
Cold/numb hands		
Active therapy	25	17
Placebo	17	14
Sexual dysfunction		
Active therapy	12	7
Placebo	6	6
Depression		
Active therapy	9	5
Placebo	6	5
Dementia		
Active therapy	2	2
Placebo	2	2

with a mean age of 71, it was apparent that a diuretic-based regimen, with a β-blocker added if necessary, reduced mortality and morbidity due to CHD in diabetic individuals.

In the SHEP study, baseline DBP was <80 mm Hg (mean, 77 mm Hg) and was reduced by treatment to <75 mm Hg in the majority of patients (mean, 68 mm Hg) without evidence of a deleterious effect on ischemic heart disease events. There was no evidence to support the concept that lowering DBP to <80-85 mm Hg would increase CHD events. But if DBP was reduced to <55-60 mm Hg, some increase in CHD events was noted. These levels, however, are rarely reached in clinical practice

In these early trials, the benefits of antihypertensive therapy were shown to be as great, or even greater, in diabetics than in nondiabetic subjects. Thiazide diuretics and β-blockers were used as baseline therapy in these studies as well as in most others prior to the mid 1990s before agents such as the ACE inhibitors, calcium channel blockers (CCBs), or ARBs became available.

In the 1970s and 1980s, it was widely publicized that the use of these agents, especially thiazide diuretics, might actually be dangerous in diabetic patients. The studies reporting this were usually retrospective case report studies with poor follow-up. After the publication of one article that suggested an increase in insulin resistance with diuretics and β-blockers, physicians were advised that these drugs should not be used in diabetics. Other comments from some investigators that the use of these agents had failed to reduce CHD events while reducing stroke and heart failure also suggested to physicians that these were not drugs of choice, especially in diabetic individuals.

A careful review of the early data, however, and the results of more trials indicate that not only are thiazide diuretics and β-blockers not harmful, they are clearly beneficial in the management of diabetic hypertensive patients. As noted in SHEP, when diabetic subjects were treated with chlorthalidone initially, with atenolol added if goal BP levels were not achieved, outcome was improved. And in the HDFP trial, mortality and morbidity were reduced significantly in the diabetic cohort. In this study, diuretics, β-blockers, hydralazine, and reserpine were the main drugs of choice. Thus physicians who were avoiding the use of these agents may have been influenced more by promotional data about the benefit of newer drugs than by results of carefully controlled, randomized, long-term treatment trials. Some trials, especially ALLHAT, have helped to clarify the role of these as well as other medications in the management of the hypertensive diabetic. In ALLHAT, the use of a diuretic-based treatment regimen resulted in similar or better CV outcome in nondiabetics as well as diabetic subjects when compared with an ACE inhibitor– or CCB-based regimen.

The question of the occurrence of hyperglycemia or new-onset diabetes (NOD) with diuretics and/or β-blockers is discussed in *Chapter 7*. On balance, it does not appear that diuretic use increases NOD by more than about 1% compared with placebo. On the other hand, β-blockers increase NOD to a greater degree. The use of an RAAS inhibitor (ACE inhibitor or ARB) as part of a therapeutic regimen results in about 2% to 5% fewer cases of NOD in hypertensive patients when compared with regimens that do not include these medications. The clinical significance of NOD has not been established (see ALLHAT results in patients with impaired fasting glucose [IFG], discussed later in this chapter).

■ **Appropriate Blood Pressure Control in Diabetes and Fosinopril vs Amlodipine Cardiovascular Event Trial**

Effects of different medications have been studied in diabetic hypertensive individuals. In the ABCD trial and FACET, the use of an ACE inhibitor, enalapril, was compared with different long-acting dihydropyridine CCBs, nisoldipine or amlodipine. In both of these studies, the use of an ACE inhibitor–based treatment program in type 2 diabetics produced a better outcome than a CCB-based treatment program (**Table 6.4** and **Table 6.5**). Fewer than 500 patients were followed in each of these trials for approximately 2 to 3 or 5 years. The total number of events was small, especially in FACET.

TABLE 6.4 — Adjusted Cardiovascular Events in the Appropriate Blood Pressure Control in Diabetes Study[a,b]

CV Event	Nisoldipine ($n=235$)	Enalapril ($n=235$)
Fatal/nonfatal MI	25[c]	5[c]
Nonfatal MI	22[c]	5[c]
Cerebrovascular accidents	11	7
CHF	6	5
Death from CV event	10	5
Death from any cause	17	13

[a] 93 Patients assigned to nisoldipine also needed a diuretic and 89 patients required a β-blocker to achieve goal BP; in the enalapril group, 99 patients required a β-blocker and 110 patients required a diuretic to achieve goal BP.
[b] 5-Year follow-up.
[c] Significant difference between groups.

Adapted from: Estacio RO, et al. *N Engl J Med.* 1998;338:645-652.

TABLE 6.5 — Cardiovascular Events in the Fosinopril vs Amlodipine Cardiovascular Events Trial[a]

CV Event	Fosinopril ($n=189$)	Amlodipine ($n=191$)
Fatal/nonfatal stroke	4	5
Fatal/nonfatal MI	10	13
Hospitalized for angina	0	4
Any major CV event	14[b]	27[b]

[a] Mean age of patients 63 years; 3.5-year follow-up.
[b] $P=0.03$.

Tatti P, et al. *Diabetes Care.* 1998;21:597-603.

Blood pressure decreases in the ABCD trial were equal with both classes of drugs, but in FACET, BP decrease was actually greater with amlodipine than with an RAAS inhibitor fosinopril (–19/8 vs –13/8 mm Hg). This has also been noted in other trials, such as the VALUE trial, in which BP lowering was greater with amlodipine (plus other medications) compared with valsartan, an ARB (plus other medications). In the VALUE trial, there were fewer MIs in patient treated with a CCB than with an ARB (possibly because of greater BP reduction).

Despite a similar or lesser degree of BP lowering when compared with the CCB, the ACE inhibitor group in both FACET and ABCD experienced fewer MIs and fewer heart failure episodes. These studies have been criticized for trial design problems and for lack of predictive power (small number of events) but appeared at the time to strengthen the argument that ACE inhibitors, usually in combination with a diuretic, were probably to be preferred to CCBs in the management of diabetic nephropathy.

What the FACET and ABCD studies did not suggest was that the use of CCBs in the management of hypertensive diabetic patients is dangerous. In FACET, outcome was improved when a CCB was added to the ACE inhibitor; benefit was greater than with the ACE inhibitor alone. Thus these studies established that CCBs might have a place in the treatment of hypertensive diabetics. These studies laid the groundwork for trials that explored specific effects of BP lowering with different medications in diabetic patients *with or without evidence of renal involvement*.

■ The United Kingdom Prospective Diabetes Study

The UKPDS was a large, prospective, randomized clinical trial. There were several facets of this trial; one was to assess the impact of intense compared with conventional glycemic control on diabetes-related and other end points. The second was to determine the effect of tight BP control compared with less effective BP control on CV events. The third was to evaluate differences in outcome with different antihypertensive regimens.

The number of type 2 diabetics recruited was 4297; of these, 1544 were hypertensive and attending hypertension clinics, 421 had previously received treatment but had BP >150/85 mm Hg, and 727 were admitted to the trial as untreated hypertensives with BP >160/90 mm Hg. The mean age was 56 years. The hypertension phase of the study recruited 1148 patients. These patients with type 2 diabetes were randomized to less-tight compared with tight BP control groups. Initial BPs were 160/94 and

159/94 mm Hg, respectively. The tight BP control group was further subdivided into patients randomly assigned to an ACE inhibitor–based regimen (captopril 25 to 50 mg bid) or to a β-blocker–based regimen (atenolol 50 to 100 mg/qd) (**Table 6.6**). Additional drug therapy included the use of furosemide (20 mg daily), a dihydropyridine calcium antagonist (nifedipine SR 10 to 40 mg bid), an α-blocker (prazosin 1 to 5 mg tid), or a centrally acting agent (α-methyldopa 250 to 500 mg bid). Medications other than ACE inhibitors or β-blockers were used in the less-tight control group.

TABLE 6.6 — Results of Different Levels of Blood Pressure Control in Hypertensive Patients With Type 2 Diabetes: β-Blocker– Compared With ACE Inhibitor–Based Treatment Program

- Better control of BP compared with less-aggressive treatment in 8.4-y follow-up of 1148 subjects (achieved BP of 144/82 mm Hg compared with 154/87 mm Hg)
- Reduced risk of:
  - Stroke (44%)
  - Fatal stroke (58%)
  - Death related to diabetes (32%)
  - HF (56%)
  - Fatal and nonfatal CHD events (21%) (trend but not significant)
- *No difference in outcome between a captopril-based and an atenolol-based treatment program*

United Kingdom Prospective Diabetes Study Group. *BMJ*. 1998;317: 703-713.

At the end of an 8½-year period, the tight BP control group (297) had achieved BP of 144/82 mm Hg compared with levels of 154/87 mm Hg in the less-tight control group (156). Thus there was a –10/–5 mm Hg difference in achieved BP. Both groups received multiple drugs in an attempt to achieve goal BP; about two thirds of the tight control group required two or more different agents; fewer patients in the less-tight cohort were on two or more drugs. This presumably reflected less of a concerted effort to lower BP. The final results of this 8½-year study are of great interest.

A difference of only –10/–5 mm Hg between the two groups of diabetic hypertensives resulted in a reduction of both macrovascular and microvascular events. Reductions of >44% in total strokes, 58% in fatal strokes, 21% in MIs, and 56% in heart failure were noted (**Table 6.6**). Diabetes-related end points were reduced overall by 24%, diabetes-related deaths by 32%, and microvascular disease (ie, retinopathy progression, loss of visual acuity, and proteinuria) by 37% (**Table 6.7**). Tighter BP control rather than the use of a specific drug regimen accounted for a dramatic decrease in both microvascular and macrovascular events. No difference in outcome was noted between the ACE inhibitor–based and the β-blocker–based groups; an important observation in view of recommendations to limit or restrict the use of β-blockers in the treatment of hypertension.

6

TABLE 6.7 — United Kingdom Prospective Diabetes Study: Effect of Blood Pressure Control on Diabetic Events

Tight BP control (144/82 mm Hg) compared with less-effective control (154/87 mm Hg)
Reduction of:
• 24% in diabetic-related end points
• 32% in deaths related to diabetes
• 37% in microvascular events, renal failure, and severe retinopathy

United Kingdom Prospective Diabetes Study Group. *BMJ*. 1998;317: 703-713.

Figure 6.3 presents specific data and risk reduction (events/1000 patient-years in the UKPDS trial). While the β-blocker group experienced more side effects and more weight gain than the ACE inhibitor group, the results of this study in 1998 at least temporarily put to rest some of the concerns about using β-blockers in patients with diabetes. It is important to note that the patients receiving β-blockers did not have an increased prevalence of hypoglycemia. Thus the concern about masking the symptoms of low blood glucose levels with a β-blocker may only be of clinical relevance in type 1 diabetic patients. Despite the results of meta-analyses that suggest that stroke

FIGURE 6.3 — Results of Tight Blood Pressure Control Compared With Less-Tight Blood Pressure Control in the United Kingdom Prospective Diabetes Study

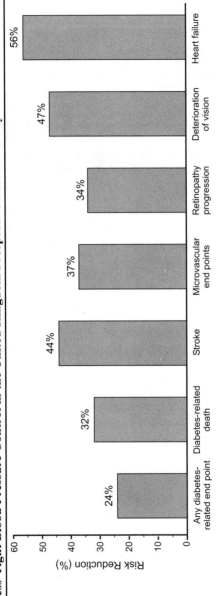

Compared with less-tight control, tight control of BP (a difference of −10/−5 mm Hg between groups) produced a 24% reduction in the risk of diabetes-related mortality, stroke, and microvascular disease ($P=0.0046$). BP control, rather than a specific treatment regimen, resulted in benefit. A combined analysis of all macrovascular diseases (including MI, SCD, stroke, and peripheral vascular disease) showed that tight control was associated with a 34% reduction risk when compared with less-tight control ($P=0.019$). All changes are statistically significant.

United Kingdom Prospective Diabetes Study Group. *BMJ.* 1998;317:703-713.

6

outcome is not as good with a β-blocker regimen as with other therapies, the use of these agents is clearly indicated in diabetic patients with angina, post MI, etc. Glycemic control in the UKPDS study was not ideal, as recently defined. HbA_{1C} was 7.2% during the first 4 years and 8.3% over 5 to 8 years. Adequate glycemic control is presently defined as an HbA_{1C} of <7%.

Despite the fact that patients did not achieve the HbA_{1C} levels that are defined as adequate control by guidelines committees, some benefit in CV outcome was noted in a long-term 10-year follow-up with patients who had the greatest decreases in HbA_{1C} levels. No difference was noted in blood glucose control between the ACE inhibitor–based and the β-blocker–based treatment groups.

■ The Captopril Prevention Project Study

Several other trials have been based on the use of an ACE inhibitor. The 5-year ACE inhibitor CAPPP study, which was a multicenter randomized, prospective, open trial but in which investigators were unaware of the occurrence of end points, included >10,000 patients with hypertension and a supine DBP >100 mm Hg. The study compared the ACE inhibitor captopril 50 to 100 mg daily (with hydrochlorothiazide and, in some cases, diltiazem added if necessary), with a regimen of a β-blocker or a diuretic or a combination of both drugs (with diltiazem added, if necessary). There are no data available on the exact number of subjects in the captopril group who required the addition of the thiazide or the number of subjects in the other treatment group who received both a β-blocker and a diuretic, but the percentage of subjects on combined therapy was high.

All-cause mortality and relative risk of CV events were similar in both groups (difference not significant). The occurrence of stroke appeared to be more common in the captopril-based nondiabetic treatment group. However, in patients with diabetes, the occurrence of MI and all fatal and cardiac events was reduced to a statistically significant greater extent in the captopril-based treatment group compared with the β-blocker–based group (**Figure 6.4** and **Table 6.8**). The incidence of NOD

FIGURE 6.4 — Comparison of Captopril–Based and β-Blocker/Diuretic–Based Therapy in Patients With Diabetes in the Captopril Prevention Project (CAPPP)

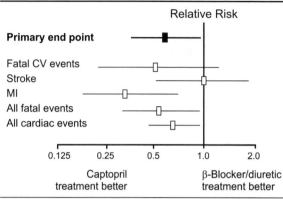

In diabetic patients, a significant reduction in all CV events, MIs, fatal events, and cardiac events was noted in the captopril-based treatment group compared with the β-blocker group. Difference in baseline characterisics may account for some of the differences in outcome.

TABLE 6.8 — Risk Reduction in Diabetic Subjects[a] in the Captopril Prevention Project

Event	Captopril vs Diuretic or β-Blocker Therapy (% Reduction)	P Value
Composite end points (fatal and nonfatal strokes and MIs)	50	0.02[b]
Stroke (fatal and nonfatal)	None	0.95
Fatal CV events	50	0.09
MIs (fatal and nonfatal)	70	0.01[b]
All CV events	30	0.03[b]

[a] $N = 572$.
[b] Statistically significant difference between the two groups of diabetic patients treated with different medications.

was also significantly lower by 14% in the captopril group. Some differences in baseline characteristics (poor randomization) may explain some of these findings, ie, initial BP was higher in the captopril group (to possibly account for more strokes in these patients), but there was a higher percentage of patients with pretreatment evidence of ischemic heart disease in the β-blocker group (which might account for some of the differences in the CHD event rates in favor of the ACE inhibitor group).

While findings in diabetics are somewhat different in the CAPPP trial from those in the UKPDS, both of these studies and data from other trials indicate that in these patients an ACE inhibitor–based treatment program will reduce CV events (except possibly stroke) to as great (or greater) degree than a β-blocker–based regimen. This is consistent with the recommendations of the Sixth and Seventh Joint National Committees (JNCs) on Prevention, Detection, Evaluation, and Treatment of High Blood Pressure that an ACE inhibitor or another RAAS inhibitor should be one component in a treatment program in hypertensive diabetics.

■ Systolic Hypertension Trial in Europe

Other trials have compared the effects of CCBs with placebo or with those of other antihypertensive medications and have included some diabetic patients. The Systolic Hypertension Trial in Europe (SYST-EUR) was a large, prospective, randomized, clinical trial designed to test the efficacy of a moderately long-acting dihydropyridine CCB, nitrendipine (not available in the United States), compared with a placebo in elderly patients with ISH and a mean age of approximately 70 years. ISH was defined as SBP >160 mm Hg with a DBP <95 mm Hg. (Values for ISH, which were being used when the study began, are no longer accepted. The new values for ISH [at least in the United States] are an SBP ≥140 and a DBP <90 mm Hg.)

There were >4600 patients randomized to placebo or active treatment, which included nitrendipine (10 to 40 mg/day) with the addition or substitution of enalapril (5 to 20 mg/day) or hydrochlorothiazide (12.5 to 25.0 mg/day) or both. Therapy was titrated to reduce SBP by

>10 mm Hg or to <150 mm Hg. Follow-up was about 2 years. The placebo-corrected decrease in BP in 4203 nondiabetic subjects was –10.3/4.5 mm Hg. In this study, there was a reduction of 42% in stroke and 26% in overall cardiac end points in treated compared with placebo subjects. This level of risk reduction is similar to that noted in the SHEP study, which used thiazide diuretics as initial therapy with β-blockers added if necessary.

There were 492 diabetic subjects, about 10% of the total number of patients in the SYST-EUR study. A BP reduction of –8.6/–3.9 mm Hg was noted in the treated diabetic hypertensive patients compared with subjects who received placebo. Overall event rates were reduced significantly in the treated patients compared with placebo subjects (**Table 6.9**). In addition, treatment of hypertension in these subjects was associated with an even greater benefit in terms of CVD risk reduction than that observed in nondiabetic patients. For example, in diabetic patients, there was a 55% reduction in total mortality compared with a 6% reduction in nondiabetics, a >70% reduction in CV mortality compared with a 13% reduction in nondiabetics, and a 69% reduction in fatal and nonfatal strokes compared with 38% in nondiabetics. All cardiac events combined were reduced by 53% compared with 26% in nondiabetics. The study concluded that the excess CVD risk and mortality usually

TABLE 6.9 — Systolic Hypertension Trial in Europe (SYST-EUR)[a]: Results in Diabetics

- BP changes—difference between therapy and placebo: –9/–4 mm Hg
- In the placebo subjects, the rate of events in diabetics was twice that in nondiabetics. Rate of events became equal in treated diabetics compared with nondiabetics
- Therapy compared with placebo:
  – Reduction of 63% in CV events
  – Reduction of 69% in strokes
  – Reduction of >70% in CV mortality

Absolute benefit was 36 compared with eight CV events/100 patient years that were prevented in diabetics and nondiabetics, respectively.

[a] Nitrendipine-based therapy.

associated with diabetics compared with nondiabetics in this elderly population was almost completely abolished by the treatment of hypertension. In this study, unlike the others previously reported, the benefit was based on the use of a longer-acting CCB as initial or baseline therapy.

It may seem counterintuitive that risk is reduced to a greater degree in diabetic hypertensive patients than in nondiabetics, but it is well known that the greater the risk and the greater the number of risk factors, the better the results of therapy. Simply stated, benefit is greatest in patients at high risk or in the elderly (who usually are at high risk with multiple risk factors). This was noted in the SHEP and UKPDS. Another major multidrug trial that used a CCB as baseline therapy (Hypertension Optimal Treatment [HOT] study) appeared to confirm that the BP goal should be set lower in diabetic patients.

■ Hypertension Optimal Treatment

The HOT study was designed to determine the optimal target BP that would result in the lowest morbidity/mortality that could be achieved in treated hypertensive patients. More than 18,000 patients from 26 European countries were randomly assigned to one of three target BP groups, <90, <85, or <80 mm Hg DBP. There were no target BP levels set for SBP. In this trial as in others, with the exception of the ISH studies (SHEP and SYST-EUR), goal BP was established only for DBP.

It has become apparent that elevated SBP is a more accurate indicator of CV risk than DBP. While most physicians will treat a patient with a persistent DBP of 95 to 100 mm Hg, many still are not treating patients with SBPs of 150 to 159 mm Hg and a normal DBP; yet, SBP at these levels poses a greater risk for CV events than DBP of 95 to 100 mm Hg (**Figure 6.5**). This may be especially true in diabetic subjects where many of the patients with type 2 diabetes are >60 years of age and have predominantly SBP elevations. Yet, as was the custom with other trials, the HOT study primarily focused on DBP. Changes in SBP were noted and considered in the final analysis of events, but these were not considered to be primary considerations.

FIGURE 6.5 — Relative Risk of Elevated Systolic and Diastolic Blood Pressure

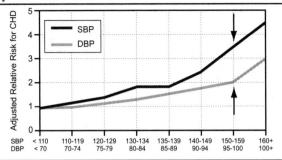

Elevated SBP may impart greater risk for CHD than elevated DBP; ie, 150-159 mm Hg SBP poses a greater risk than 95-100 mm Hg DBP. *See text.*

Data from: Multiple Risk Factor Intervention Trial Research Group. *JAMA*. 1990;263:1795-1801.

In the HOT study, DBP levels were titrated using the dihydropyridine CCB felodipine as primary therapy, with other drugs added as necessary; these included ACE inhibitors, β-blockers, and thiazide diuretics. In many cases, three or more medications were necessary to achieve goal BP. One of the reasons for this may have been that diuretics were only added after the other drugs had been titrated upward. It is quite possible that more subjects would have responded to fewer medications if a diuretic had been added as a second step. Patients were followed for approximately 4 years and the impact of different levels of achieved BP on CV events was recorded. The lowest incidence of major CV events occurred with a mean SBP of 139 mm Hg and a DBP of 83 mm Hg. Lowest CV mortality was noted at levels of 139/87 mm Hg. Most of the benefit therefore occurred in patients who achieved BP <140/90 mm Hg, a level consistent with the recommendations of most US and international guidelines for a majority of hypertensive individuals.

Within the HOT study, there were 1501 (8%) diabetic subjects. Among all of the patients in the HOT study, there was little difference in overall morbidity/mortality between those who achieved <90 mm Hg, <85 mm Hg, or <80 mm Hg DBP (actual achieved BPs in the three target groups were 85, 83, and 81 mm Hg) (**Figure 6.6**). However, within the diabetic group, there was a significant difference between groups. There was a 51%

FIGURE 6.6 — Patients With Diabetes in the Hypertension Optimal Treatment Study

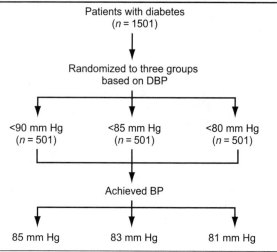

Hansson L, et al. *Lancet*. 1998;351:1755-1762.

reduction in CV events and a reduction of 43% in CV mortality in hypertensive diabetic patients who achieved a target BP of ≤80 mm Hg compared with those in the <90 mm Hg cohort (**Figure 6.7**). Targets achieved were 140/81 mm Hg compared with 144/85 mm Hg, a difference of only –4/–4 mm Hg. Thus this trial, as well as the MD Renal Disease and the UKPDS, indicates that targeting lower BP in diabetics than in nondiabetics is beneficial. These observations are consistent with the idea that diabetic subjects have an increased tendency toward vascular injury when BP is even slightly elevated and that reducing BP to as close to the normotensive range or ideal BP of 120/80 mm Hg is a goal to be achieved if at all possible. Again, the JNCs, the National Kidney Foundation, and the American Diabetes Association (ADA) recommendations for lower BP goals in diabetics seem reasonable.

FIGURE 6.7 — Cardiovascular Events in Diabetics in the Hypertension Optimal Treatment Study

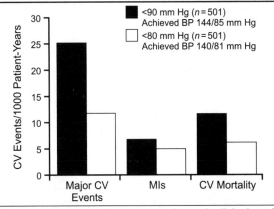

CV events were reduced to a greater degree in diabetics who achieved the lowest levels of DBP (difference in BP –4/–4 mm Hg).

Modified from: Hansson L, et al. *Lancet.* 1998;351:1755-1762.

In the HOT study, the use of aspirin proved beneficial in reducing CHD events in diabetic patients as well as in the rest of the study population. There appears to be potential benefit and little danger with aspirin therapy in hypertensive subjects *if their BP is controlled.*

The HOT study, as well as the UKPDS, pointed out the need to rethink our approach to the diabetic patient and to emphasize that management of hypertension may be as or more important than glycemic control in these patients. Thus the emphasis should shift from glycemic control *alone* to a more multifaceted approach. There was no evidence in the diabetic cohort in the HOT study or in other trials, such as UKPDS or SYST-EUR, to suggest that aggressive treatment is harmful or that it increases MI or ischemic heart disease events. Although the concept of the J-curve is an interesting one (ie, that reducing DBP <80-85 mm Hg might actually increase the number of ischemic heart disease events in patients with plaque formation or previous ischemic heart disease), there is little evidence that there may be an adverse effect before

DBP levels decrease to <55-60 mm Hg. As noted, these lower levels are infrequently achieved in clinical practice.

Both the HOT and the SHEP studies suggest that decreasing DBP to <80 mm Hg is not only safe but may actually decrease the number of ischemic heart disease events. Many physicians are concerned about treating the elderly diabetic patient with ISH because of concern about decreasing DBP too much. Again, the HOT study, as well as others, seems to have put that fear to rest. Many diabetics >65 years of age will have BP of 150-180/80-85 mm Hg. Decreasing the SBP to more normal levels is clearly beneficial, even if the DBP decreases to levels of 70-75 mm Hg.

It is important to note that *most of the medications that are currently in use decrease SBP to a greater degree than DBP and reduce pulse pressure.* An increased pulse pressure is indicative of increased vascular rigidity, an important prognostic indicator of increased risk. There are no data yet to indicate that decreasing pulse pressure improves prognosis, but a decrease may indicate some decrease in vessel rigidity that may be beneficial. There is no reason why a patient with or without diabetes with elevated SBP with normal DBP should not have their BP reduced.

The well-controlled, randomized clinical trials, which now have included >8000 diabetic hypertensive patients, have clearly indicated that lowering BP is beneficial; morbidity and mortality, not just from macrovascular but also from microvascular events, will be reduced. The clinical trials in diabetic patients reported to date indicate that it is possible to reduce BP to goal levels or near goal levels of 130/80-85 mm Hg in many but not all patients with the available antihypertensive medications with or without lifestyle interventions. It is obvious from these trials that more than one medication is often required. In fact, in diabetic patients, there is some evidence to suggest that the use of a combination of drugs as initial therapy, eg, an ACE inhibitor and a diuretic, an ARB/diuretic combination, an ACE inhibitor/CCB combination, or in some instances, a β-blocker/diuretic combination, might be appropriate.

■ Heart Outcome Prevention Evaluation

The HOPE study included a large number of diabetic subjects. This was not primarily a trial of patients with hypertension since the average BP prior to entering the trial was 139/79 mm Hg. In this trial, 3577 high-risk patients with diabetes with a mean age >55 years were included. A large majority had multiple risk factors or evidence of ischemic heart disease. Most patients were on multiple drugs for either hypertension or other diseases prior to entering the trial. No patients with clinical proteinuria, heart failure, or low ejection fraction or patients who were taking ACE inhibitors were included in the study. Patients, most of whom were already on multiple medications, were randomly assigned an ACE inhibitor (ramipril 10 mg/day) given at night or placebo. The study was stopped 6 months prematurely after 4 to 5 years because of a consistent benefit in the ACE-inhibitor group compared with the control subjects who were not receiving an ACE inhibitor. As noted elsewhere, the risk of the combined primary outcome was reduced by 25%, MI by 22%, stroke by 33%, CV death by 37%, total mortality by 27%, revascularization by 17%, and overt nephropathy by 24% in the group that received the ACE inhibitor (**Table 6.10**). Primary outcome events were reduced by 25% after adjusting for the changes in SBP and DBP. These were minimal; BPs in the ACE group were only 2-4/1 mm Hg lower than in the other group. The CV benefit

TABLE 6.10 — Results of the Heart Outcome Prevention Evaluation Study in Diabetes[a]

Event	Reduction in Risk[b]
Combined primary outcome	↓ 25%
MI	↓ 22%
Stroke	↓ 33%
CV death	↓ 37%
Total mortality	↓ 27%
Overt nephropathy	↓ 24%

[a] Number of patients studied 3577, age >55 years.

[b] ACE inhibitor group compared with subjects not receiving an ACE inhibitor. The use of this agent in addition to other medications reduced CV events.

appeared to be greater than that attributable to the slight decrease in BP. A study of ambulatory BP monitoring in a small subset of HOPE patients reported a greater decrease in nighttime BP than in control subjects. Thus some of the benefits might be attributable to the changes in nocturnal BP and 24-hour BP load. In this high-risk group of diabetic patients, the benefit of treatment could have resulted from specific effects of blockade of the RAAS.

As noted in *Chapter 5*, blockade of the RAAS has proved to be useful in diabetic patients, not only in improving nephropathy especially in patients with proteinuria but in reducing some of the basic physiologic changes that are noted in the diabetic—specifically, endothelial dysfunction, which is the hallmark of the atherosclerotic process. The HOPE study, therefore, suggests that in high-risk diabetic patients, even in the absence of significant elevations of BP, the use of an ACE inhibitor as part of the program may not only be beneficial in reducing complications but in reducing other adverse events. Studies also suggest that the use of an ARB when added to other therapies will result in similar levels of CVD event reduction.

■ The HOPE/HOPE-TOO Study

This trial was an extension of the HOPE study. The objectives were to assess whether the benefits of the ACE inhibitor ramipril observed during the initial HOPE trial were maintained after trial cessation during an additional 2.6 years of follow-up. A total of 4528 of the original 9297 patients agreed to further follow-up. The proportions of patients with diabetes were similar during the main study and the extension phase (38.5% and 38.4%, respectively). The rates of ramipril and placebo use during the follow-up phase were also similar to those during the primary study. During posttrial follow-up, patients treated with the ACE inhibitor had an additional 19% lower relative risk (RR) of MI, a 16% lower RR of revascularization, and a 34% lower RR of a new diagnosis of diabetes (**Figure 6.8**). Similar RR reductions in vascular events were observed during and after the active phase of the trial, regardless of baseline CV risk level or other treatments. The results of this study suggest that the

FIGURE 6.8 — Kaplan-Meier Estimates for Outcome of Development of Diabetes: HOPE-TOO

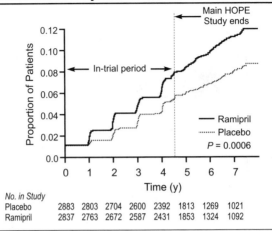

No. in Study								
Placebo	2883	2803	2704	2600	2392	1813	1269	1021
Ramipril	2837	2763	2672	2587	2431	1853	1324	1092

Kaplan-Meier estimates for the outcome of the development of diabetes in the ramipril and placebo groups in the centers continuing in the study extension.

HOPE/HOPE-TOO Study Investigators. *Circulation*. 2005;112:1339-1346.

benefits of continuing treatment with an ACE inhibitor as part of a treatment regimen in patients with varying levels of CV risk are maintained over the long term.

■ Losartan Intervention for Endpoint Reduction in Hypertension

The Losartan Intervention for Endpoint Reduction in Hypertension (LIFE) study demonstrated a significant reduction in strokes and in the development of diabetes in a group of hypertensive patients with LVH who were treated with an ARB-based (losartan) regimen when compared with patients on a β-blocker–based (atenolol) program (see *Chapter 5* and *Chapter 7* for differences in NOD between groups). In addition, in a diabetic subgroup treated with ARB-based therapy, CV events were reduced to a greater extent than in nondiabetics (**Figure 6.9**).

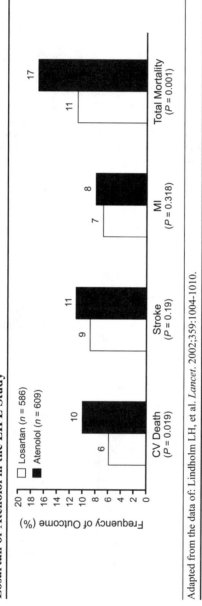

FIGURE 6.9 — Clinical Outcomes Among Diabetic Hypertensives Treated With Losartan or Atenolol in the LIFE Study

Adapted from the data of: Lindholm LH, et al. *Lancet.* 2002;359:1004-1010.

114

■ The Antihypertensive and Lipid-Lowering Treatment to Prevent Heart Attack Trial

ALLHAT was a large, randomized, double-blind, controlled trial in hypertensive patients ≥55 years of age with at least 1 other CV risk factor. This is the only large clinical trial comparing different therapies that was double-blinded; other trials, such as Anglo-Scandinavian Cardiac Outcomes Trial (ASCOT), VALUE, and LIFE, were not blinded to medications given. One reported pre-specified substudy sought to determine whether first-step antihypertensive drug therapy with an ACE inhibitor or a CCB would provide better protection against CVD events than diuretic therapy in 31,512 hypertensive patients stratified into three groups; people with DM, IFG, or normoglycemic (NG) individuals. Patients were randomized to initial treatment with chlorthalidone (12.5 to 25 mg/day), amlodipine (2.5 to 10 mg/day), or lisinopril (10 to 40 mg/day). After a mean follow-up of 4.9 years, there was no significant difference in RR for the primary outcome (fatal CHD or nonfatal MI) in DM or NG patients assigned to amlodipine or lisinopril compared with chlorthalidone or in IFG participants assigned to lisinopril compared with chlorthalidone. A significantly higher RR (RR, 1.73) was noted, however, for the primary outcome in IFG patients assigned to amlodipine compared with chlorthalidone.

Stroke was more common in NG patients assigned to lisinopril compared with chlorthalidone. Heart failure was more common in DM and NG patients assigned to amlodipine or lisinopril than in patients taking chlorthalidone (**Figure 6.10**). In the DM group, SBP was significantly lower throughout follow-up in patients assigned to chlorthalidone compared with amlodipine (1- to 2-mm Hg difference) or lisinopril (2- to 3-mm Hg difference). DBP was significantly lower in the DM participants assigned to amlodipine compared with chlorthalidone (approximately 1-mm Hg difference). There was a similar but less consistent pattern for differences in SBP and DBP between the treatment groups in the NG stratum. There was no consistently significant difference in SBP or DBP across the three treatment groups for the IFG patients. The investigators concluded that the results indicated

FIGURE 6.10 — ALLHAT Study: Coronary Heart Disease for Patients With Impaired Fasting Glucose Level at Baseline

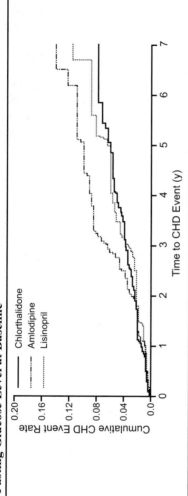

No difference lisinopril/chlorthalidone (*P*=0.56); significant difference amlodipine/chlorathalidone (*P*=0.02).

Modified from: Whelton PK, et al. *Arch Intern Med.* 2005;165:1401-1409.

no evidence of superiority for treatment with CCBs or ACE inhibitors compared with a thiazide-type diuretic as initial antihypertensive therapy in patients with diabetes, IFG, or in subjects who were normoglycemic (see *Chapter 7*, under the section *New-Onset Diabetes With Antihypertensive Medications*, and **Figures 7.2** and **7.3**).

■ The Anglo-Scandinavian Cardiac Outcomes Trial—Blood Pressure–Lowering Arm

The Anglo-Scandinavian Cardiac Outcomes Trial—Blood Pressure–Lowering Arm (ASCOT-BPLA) trial was designed to compare the effects of two treatment algorithms—amlodipine as initial therapy with added perindopril as required or atenolol with added bendroflumethiazide and potassium as required—on the incidence of various CV events, primarily nonfatal MI and fatal CHD. A total of 19,257 patients with hypertension who were 40-79 years of age and had at least three other CV risk factors were enrolled in this nonblinded study. Of these, 5145 (27%) had diabetes, a prespecified subgroup that was randomized to the two treatment arms. The study was stopped prematurely after 5.5 years' median follow-up. In the total patient population, fewer individuals on the amlodipine-based regimen had a primary end point compared with those on the atenolol-based regimen (429 vs 474, respectively), although the difference was not significant ($P=0.1052$). The total number of cardiovascular events and procedures (a secondary end point) in the diabetic subgroup was significantly lower with the amlodipine-based regimen compared with the atenolol-based regimen (430 vs 493; $P=0.0283$) (**Figure 6.11**).

As in the VALUE study, the BP decrease was greater during the titration phase (first few months) with amlodipine than with the β-blocker. Some investigators believe this early decrease in BP may at least partially explain the better outcome. They believed that in general it is the degree of BP lowering and level achieved that accounts for the improvements in CV outcome rather than the specific medications used. At the end of the study, 53% of all patients had reached both the SBP and DBP targets. While 60% of nondiabetic patients achieved target BP, only 32% of patients with diabetes reached

FIGURE 6.11 — ASCOT-BPLA: Effect of Treatment on Primary and Secondary End Points

	Amlodipine-Based Regimen (n = 9639)		Atenolol-Based Regimen (n = 9618)		
	Number (%)	Rate per 1000	Number (%)	Rate per 1000	Unadjusted HR (95% CI)
Primary Endpoints					
Nonfatal MI (including silent) + fatal CHD	429 (5)	8.2	474 (5)	9.1	0.90 (0.79-1.02)
Secondary Endpoints					
Nonfatal MI	390 (4)	7.4	444 (5)	8.5	0.87 (0.76-1.00)
Total coronary endpoint	753 (8)	14.6	852 (9)	16.8	0.87 (0.79-0.96)
Total CV events and procedures	1362 (14)	27.4	1602 (17)	32.8	0.84 (0.78-0.90)
All-cause mortality	738 (8)	13.9	820 (9)	15.5	0.89 (0.81-0.99)
CV mortality	263 (3)	4.9	342 (4)	6.5	0.76 (0.65-0.90)
Fatal and nonfatal stroke	327 (3)	6.2	422 (4)	8.1	0.77 (0.66-0.89)
Fatal and nonfatal HF	134 (1)	2.5	159 (2)	3.0	0.84 (0.66-1.05)

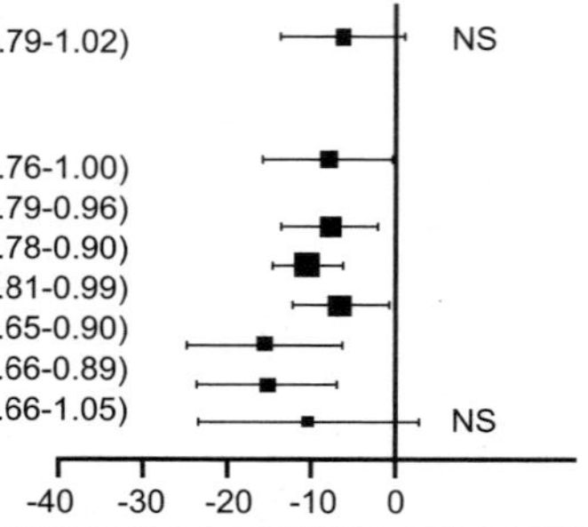

Modified from: Dahlof B, et al. *Lancet.* 2005;366:895-906.

their goals. It is interesting to note that the incidence of developing diabetes was less on the amlodipine-based regimen (567 vs 799, respectively; $P <0.0001$).

Treatment of Diabetic Nephropathy

In the 1990s, a series of studies focused on the treatment of diabetic nephropathy, primarily in type 1 diabetes. The main objective of these trials was to determine whether the use of an ACE inhibitor–based treatment program compared with a regimen that did not include an ACE inhibitor would have a beneficial impact on urinary albumin excretion rates as a surrogate of progression of diabetic nephropathy and the occurrence of renal failure. In addition, data on the necessity for dialysis and transplantation were accumulated.

Most of the trials were actually trials of multiple-drug therapy, as were earlier and later studies. For example, in one early trial, The Effect of an Angiotensin-Converting Enzyme Inhibitor on Diabetic Nephropathy, >75% of patients in the ACE inhibitor group were also receiving thiazide diuretics and β-blockers; these additional medications were necessary to reduce BP to as close to goal as possible. The other treatment group received multiple medications, but they did not include an ACE inhibitor. A significant decrease in morbidity/mortality and less progression to renal failure, dialysis, and transplantation were noted in the ACE inhibitor–treated patients (**Table 6.11**).

TABLE 6.11 — Major Outcome Events in Patients With Type 1 Diabetes and Nephropathy

| Event | Other Medications (N) | |
	With ACE-I	Without ACE-I
Death	8	14
Dialysis or transplantation	20	31
Doubling of serum creatinine	23	42
Hyperkalemia	3	0

Key: ACE-I, angiotensin-converting enzyme inhibitor.

Lewis EJ, et al. *N Engl J Med*. 1993;329:1456.

There were only minor differences in achieved BP between the two groups. One problem with this trial was that the control group subjects had significantly more proteinuria at baseline (3 g/day) compared with the ACE group (2.5 g/day). Since the degree of proteinuria is predictive of the stage of renal function deterioration, it is possible that the non–ACE-treated group had more renal disease at baseline than the ACE-treated group (**Table 6.12**). This could have affected results.

Similar benefits have been reported when BP was lowered in type 1 diabetics with nephropathy with a combination of thiazide diuretics, β-blockers, and hydralazine. These data indicate that lowering BP with multiple medications, one of which decreases the activity of the RAAS, results in slowing down progression of renal disease (β-blockers decrease the generation of renin; ACE inhibitors block conversion to angiotensin II; and while ARBs do not decrease production of angiotensin II, they block its action at the receptor site).

Numerous studies with ACE inhibitors and ARBs have confirmed that either of these agents should be part of the treatment regimen in diabetic nephropathy, especially if proteinuria is present; that there may be beneficial effects on renal function in diabetics independent of effects on BP. Renovascular resistance is decreased by ACE inhibition; blockade of the RAAS may also improve endothelial dysfunction, the propensity toward early atherogenesis, and smooth muscle hypertrophy, all factors noted in diabetic and hypertensive patients. As noted, studies with ARBs also suggest that the use of these agents will decrease CV morbidity and mortality. The clinical trials with these agents have clearly established their role in the management of type 2 diabetic patients with nephropathy (RENAAL, IDNT, and IRMA 2 trial).

The results of these three trials, RENAAL, IDNT, and IRMA 2, have helped to clarify the role of ARBs in the management of the diabetic patient with varying degrees of renal disease. A recent study (ONTARGET) concluded that an ARB was as effective as an ACE inhibitor as monotherapy with fewer side effects (ie, less cough) but did not report additional benefit when an ARB (telmisartan) and an ACE inhibitor (ramipril) were

TABLE 6.12 — Baseline Characteristics of Patients With Diabetic Nephropathy in the Captopril and Placebo Groups

Characteristic	Captopril ($n=207$)	Placebo ($n=202$)	P Value
Hypertensive (%)	75	74	0.91
On antihypertensive therapy (%)	60	59	0.84
SBP	137	140	0.21
DBP	85	86	0.47
Serum creatinine (mg/dL)	1.3	1.3	—
24-h urinary protein excretion (mg/d)	2500 ± 2500	3000 ± 2600	0.02[a]

[a] Statistically significant difference.

Lewis EJ, et al. *N Engl J Med.* 1993;329:1456.

given together compared with the use of an ACE inhibitor alone. More adverse reactions, such as hypotension, were noted with combination therapy.

■ Reduction of Endpoints in NIDDM With an Angiotensin II Antagonist, Losartan

RENAAL was a 3-year, multinational controlled trial evaluating the effects on renal function of an ARB, losartan (Cozaar) 50-100 mg/day, when added to other medications in 1513 type 2 diabetic patients. The group on losartan was compared with similar patients whose therapy included antihypertensive medications other than an ACE inhibitor or an ARB (the "placebo" group). Patients had average baseline BP of 153/82 mm Hg with evidence of diabetic nephropathy with proteinuria (>500 mg/day) and mean baseline creatinine levels of 1.9 mg/dL. At the end of the trial, there was a significant reduction in the risk of renal disease progression with fewer patients requiring renal dialysis or transplantation in the ARB group compared with the non–ARB-treated group. This was the first study to specifically demonstrate a statistically significant decrease in progression to ESRD in patients with type 2 diabetic nephropathy. A 16% reduction in the composite end point, doubling of serum creatinine, ESRD, and death was noted. A 28% ($P=0.002$) decrease in the occurrence of ESRD was noted in the group of patients treated with losartan (**Figure 6.12**). Studies with ACE inhibitor–based therapy had previously reported a reduction in progression of proteinuria in these patients but not a significant reduction in ESRD. No difference in mortality or the total number of CV events (a secondary end point) was noted, but 32% ($P=0.005$) fewer episodes of hospitalization for congestive heart failure occurred in the group receiving the ARB compared with patients who were treated with other agents.

■ Irbesartan in Diabetic Nephropathy Trial

IDNT compared results of treatment of three groups of subjects with type 2 diabetes, significant proteinuria, and evidence of renal functional impairment. One thousand seven hundred fifteen patients were randomized to

FIGURE 6.12 — Kaplan-Meier Curve of the Percentage of Type 2 Diabetic Patients With End-Stage Renal Disease in the RENAAL Study

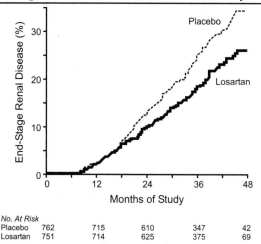

Losartan graph line indicates therapy with ARB plus other medications, while the placebo line shows therapy with medications other than an ARB or ACE inhibitor. (RR, 28%; *P*=0.002.)

Brenner BM, et al. *N Engl J Med*. 2001;345:865.

receive 1) an ARB, irbesartan (Avapro), up to 300 mg/ qd, in addition to medications other than an ACE inhibitor or a CCB; or 2) amlodipine 2.5-10 mg/qd in addition to other medications other than the study drugs; or 3) medications other than the study drugs (a so-called placebo group).

Mean duration of the study was 2.6 years. Primary end point of the study was a composite end point of development of ESRD, death from any cause, and the time to doubling of the serum creatinine concentration (**Figure 6.13**). Treatment with irbesartan plus other medications that did not include an ACE inhibitor, another ARB, or a CCB resulted in a significant 20% reduction in risk of the primary end point and 33% reduction in the risk of doubling of serum creatinine within the trial period compared with patients treated with medications other than an ACE inhibitor, ARB, or CCB (the "placebo"

FIGURE 6.13 — Cumulative Proportions of Patients Reaching Primary End Points[a] in the IDNT

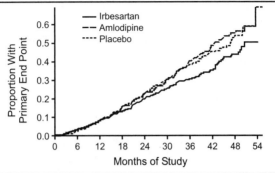

Proportion of patients with primary end points. Differences between irbesartan and placebo and irbesartan and amlodipine were significant (–20% [$P=0.02$] and –23% [$P=0.006$], respectively).

[a] Doubling of baseline serum creatinine, end-stage renal disease, and death from any cause.

Lewis EJ, et al. *N Engl J Med.* 2001;345:856.

group). Of interest was the finding of a 23% reduction ($P=0.006$) in the primary end point and a 37% reduction ($P=0.001$) in risk of doubling of creatinine in the irbesartan group compared with subjects on a regimen based on amlodipine (plus other medications except ARBs and ACE inhibitors). Achieved BP differences between the ARB and CCB group were not significant. Proteinuria was also significantly reduced in the irbesartan group compared with other therapies. No difference in all-cause mortality was noted among groups in this trial. This trial provides some additional evidence to suggest a better outcome in patients with diabetes and renal disease who are treated with an RAAS inhibitor compared with those on a CCB-based regimen.

- **Irbesartan Microalbuminura Type 2 Diabetes Mellitus in Hypertension Patients**

  The IRMA 2 trial compared the effects on patients of irbesartan (150 or 300 mg/day) plus other medications (other than ACE inhibitors or ARBs) with patients on medications other than an ARB or ACE inhibitor. Five hundred ninety type 2 diabetic patients who demonstrated microproteinuria (30-300 mg/day) were followed for 2 years. No significant differences in achieved BP were noted in the three groups of patients. There was, however, a 70% reduction in progression to more severe renal disease in the group of patients treated with irbesartan; doses of 300 mg proved to be more effective than the 150-mg dose. The group that received irbesartan 300 mg/day compared with the non-ARB group experienced a significant reduction in the number who progressed to frank proteinuria (>300 mg/day). In addition, 34% normalized the amount of albumin excreted (**Figure 6.14**).

FIGURE 6.14 — Progression of Diabetic Nephropathy in IRMA 2 Study of Hypertensive Patients With Type 2 Diabetes and Microproteinuria

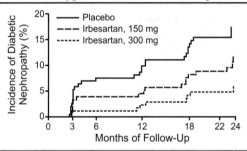

Progression of diabetic nephropathy in the IRMA 2 study of hypertensive patients with type 2 diabetes and microproteinuria. Placebo represents medications other than an ARB or ACE inhibitor. In the irbesartan 150-mg and 300-mg groups, a medication other than another ARB or ACE inhibitor can be given. The difference between placebo and 150-mg irbesartan was not significant ($P = 0.08$); between placebo and 300-mg irbesartan, $P < 0.001$.

Parving HH, et al. *N Engl J Med*. 2001;345:875.

■ **Overview: Role of ARBs**

In all of the described trials, the ACE inhibitor or ARB used was well tolerated. The results of these studies, including ONTARGET, have important treatment implications and suggest that recommendations for treatment of hypertension in type 2 diabetics (which previously included the use of ACE inhibitors as a preferred treatment) now include the use of ARBs as well, especially in diabetic nephropathy with proteinuria. As previously noted, one of the trials (IDNT) indicated that renal disease progression can be delayed to a greater extent with an ARB than with a CCB-based treatment program. In all cases, however, multiple medications will usually be necessary to achieve goal BP; treatment should include the use of a diuretic.

Data indicate that not only can the progression to more severe renal disease be slowed by the use of an ARB, but that signs of glomerular dysfunction, ie, proteinuria, may be improved with a decrease in microproteinuria. These findings are similar to those regarding LVH in hypertension. LVH can be regressed with treatment or actually prevented if BP is lowered in hypertensive individuals before LVH becomes apparent.

Clinical Uncertainties in Treatment Decisions in Hypertensive Diabetics

A major problem with the management of the diabetic hypertensive occurs when physicians, who have been advised to reduce BP in these patients to <130/80-85 mmHg instead of to <140/90 mmHg as in nondiabetics, do not optimize therapy. In about 50% of diabetic hypertensives, therapy is not changed when BP is still above present guideline levels. For example, in patients with office BP <140/90 mmHg but higher than recommended levels of 130/80-85 mmHg for home, medications may not be changed. Uncertainty by the provider about the levels of BP that might be most effective in reducing CV events may play a role in the lack of achievement of goal BP levels. This is in addition to problems relating to multiple comorbidities in the diabetic population and the lack of urgency in lowering BP.

The SANDS Study: Lower BP and Lipid Goals—Better Results?

A recent trial, the Stop Atherosclerosis in Native Diabetics Study (SANDS) in type 2 diabetics, examined the effects of intensive reduction of BP with a regimen based initially on an ACE inhibitor and diuretic and later with an ARB plus a diuretic, with a goal of <115/75 mmHg in one group compared with 130/80 mm Hg in another. In addition, aggressive reduction of LDL to a target of 70 mg/dL with statin therapy was also attempted in a native American Indian population. Lower BP levels than those currently recommended were safely achieved in men and women with type 2 diabetes (achieved BP in the aggressive group was 116/67 mm Hg compared with BP in the standard group of 128/73 mmHg). The SBP goal of 115 mmHg was associated with a reduction in carotid intimal thickness and a greater reduction in left ventricular mass when compared with standard treatments. There were no measurable differences in the small number of CV events. Thus it appears that lower BP and lipid goals can be achieved, at least in this population, and that risk markers for CV disease can be reduced by intensive therapy.

6

Summary

The results of key hypertension treatment trials in diabetic patients are summarized in **Table 6.13**. It is important to note that there is a trend favoring the use of an ACE inhibitor/diuretic or an ARB/diuretic combination in diabetic patients, despite treatment results with a β-blocker/diuretic regimen in the UKPDS trial. This latter approach is probably not preferred treatment. Based on recent data, a regimen with an ACE inhibitor or an ARB rather than one based on CCB therapy is preferred in diabetic patients, but in most cases, a multiple drug regimen is necessary to lower BP to goal levels. An ACE inhibitor or an ARB plus a CCB is also a reasonable and effective approach.

It is also clear that better BP control results in better outcome. Outcome is improved in both young and older diabetics to a great or greater degree than in nondiabetics. These trials have answered many questions that were posed several years ago before the trials were completed (**Table 6.14**). There are now enough data available to indicate vigorous treatment of diabetic patients with hypertension.

TABLE 6.13 — Randomized Controlled Clinical Trials of Antihypertensive Therapy in Type 2 Diabetic Patients With Hypertension

Trial (N)	Treatment (n)	F/U (y)	BP Decrease SBP/DPB (mm Hg)	End Points	Risk Reduction: Therapy vs Control (%)
Comparative Trials					
ABCD (470)	Nisoldipine	2	20/10	Death from CV events	Enalapril vs nisoldipine: −51
	Enalapril		20/10 (estimated from graph)		
ALLHAT		4.9		Fatal CHD or nonfatal MI	No significant difference in RR for the primary outcome in DM or NG participants assigned to amlodipine or lisinopril vs chlorthalidone or in IFG vs chlorthalidone or participants assigned to lisinopril vs chlorthalidone
Diabetic (13,101)	Chlorthalidone		8/10		
	Amlodipine		10/9		
	Lisinopril		9/9		
IFG (1399)	Chlorthalidone		14/11		
	Amlodipine		13/10		
	Lisinopril		12/10		
NG (17,012)	Chlorthalidone		13/9		
	Amlodipine		13/10		
	Lisinopril		12/9		

Study	Treatment (n)	Follow-up (y)		End point	Results
ASCOT-BLM Diabetic (5145)	Amlodipine ± perindopril (2567)	5.5	Not reported	Nonfatal MI (including silent MI) plus fatal CHD (secondary end point)	Not reported
	Atenolol ± thiazide (2578)			Total CV events and procedures	Amlodipine vs atenolol: –13%
CAPPP (632)	Captopril + diuretic or CCB	6	10/10 (estimated from graph)	Fatal or nonfatal MI; all CV events	Captopril vs conventional treatment: MIs: –66 CV events: –33
	β-Blocker or thiazide ± CCB				
FACET (380)	Fosinopril (189)	3.5	13/8	Combined MI, stroke, or hospitalized angina	Fosinopril vs amlodipine: –51
	Amlodipine (191)		19/8		
LIFE (1195) Diabetic	Losartan (586)	4.7	17/11	Composite of CV morbidity and mortality	Losartan vs atenolol: –24 (CV death, stroke, or MI)
	Atenolol (609)		19/11		
MIDAS (425)	Isradipine	3	18/13	CVD events	Isradipine (5.65) vs HCTZ (3.17)
	HCTZ		19/13		

Continued

TABLE 6.13 — *Continued*

Trial (N)	Treatment (n)	F/U (y)	BP Decrease SBP/DPB (mm Hg)	End Points	Risk Reduction: Therapy vs Control (%)
Isolated Systolic Hypertension Trials					
SHEP (583)	Chlorthalidone + atenolol or reserpine Placebo	5	Active vs placebo: 9.6/2.2	Major CVD events Major CHD events Nonfatal MI, fatal MI Strokes	−34 −56 −54 −22
SYST- EUR (492)	Nitrendipine + enalapril or HCTZ (252) Placebo (240)	2	Active vs placebo: 10.1/4.5	CVD mortality CVD events Strokes	−76 −63 −73
BP Control: Tight vs Less-Tight					
HOT (1501) Diabetic	Felodipine + ACE-I + β-blocker + diuretic: DBP <90 mm Hg DBP <85 mm Hg DBP <80 mm Hg	4-5	26.2/20.3 28.0/22.3 29.3/24.3	Major CVD events CVD mortality Total mortality	(Risk increases in <90 vs <80 group) +100 +200 +77

UKPDS (1148)	Tight vs less-tight BP control (390)	8	10/5	Diabetes-related end point −24
				Diabetes-related deaths −32
				Strokes −44
				Microvascular events −37
	β-Blocker[a] (358) ACE-I program (400)	8		No significant difference between treatment groups

Key: ACE-I, angiotensin-converting enzyme inhibitor; F/U, follow-up; DM, diabetes mellitus; NG, normoglycemic.

Trials strongly suggest that strict control of BP in diabetics is beneficial and that a medication that decreases the activity of the RAAS should be part of the treatment regimen.

[a] Number to treat to prevent one event: 15.

TABLE 6.14 — Answers Provided by the Treatment Trials in Diabetics With Hypertension

- Lowering BP in hypertensive diabetics reduces CV morbidity and mortality: risk reduction is greater than in nondiabetics
- Continuous lowering of BP may be more effective than improving glycemic control
- Lowering BP will also delay progression of retinopathy and nephropathy
- Patients should be treated if BP is >140/90 mm Hg
- Goal for treated BP should be set at ≤130/80-85 mm Hg
- Treatment programs based on ACE inhibitors, ARBs, diuretics, β-blockers, and CCBs have produced beneficial results; the use of an ACE inhibitor–based regimen may be more effective in reducing CV events than a CCB–based treatment program, especially in patients with nephropathy
- A treatment regimen that includes an ARB compared with a program without an ARB or ACE inhibitor significantly reduces progression of renal disease in patients with type 2 diabetes
- Most hypertensive diabetics will require multiple medications to achieve goal BP; therapy should include an ACE inhibitor or an ARB, usually with a diuretic, or an ACE inhibitor or ARB and CCB

SELECTED READING

Bosch J, Lonn E, Pogue J, et al; HOPE/HOPE-TOO Study Investigators. Long-term effects of ramipril on cardiovascular events and on diabetes: results of the HOPE study extension. *Circulation.* 2005;112:1339-1346.

Brenner BM, Cooper ME, de Zeeuw, et al for the RENAAL Study Investigators. Effects of losartan on renal and cardiovascular outcomes in patients with type 2 diabetes and nephropathy. *N Engl J Med.* 2001; 345:861-869.

Chowdhury TA, Kumar S, Barnett AH, Dodson PM. Treatment of hypertension in patients with type 2 diabetes: a review of the recent evidence. *J Hum Hypertens.* 1999;13:803-811.

Curb JD, Pressel SL, Cutler JA, et al. Effect of diuretic-based antihypertensive treatment on cardiovascular disease risk in older diabetic patients with isolated systolic hypertension. Systolic Hypertension in the Elderly Program Cooperative Research Group. *JAMA.* 1996;276:1886-1892.

Dahlof B, Sever PS, Poulter NR, et al; ASCOT Investigators. Prevention of cardiovascular events with an antihypertensive regimen of amlodipine adding perindopril as required versus atenolol adding bendroflumethiazide as required, in the Anglo-Scandinavian Cardiac Outcomes Trial-Blood Pressure Lowering Arm (ASCOT-BPLA): a multicentre randomized controlled trial. *Lancet.* 2005;366:895-906.

Estacio RO, Jeffers BW, Hiatt WR, Biggerstaff SL, Gifford N, Schrier RW. The effect of nisoldipine as compared with enalapril on cardiovascular outcomes in patients with non–insulin-dependent diabetes and hypertension. *N Engl J Med.* 1998;338:645-652.

Hansson L, Lindholm LH, Ekborn T, et al. Randomized trial of old and new antihypertensive drugs in elderly patients. Cardiovascular morbidity and mortality in the Swedish Trial in Older Patients with Hypertension-2 study. *Lancet.* 1999;354:1751-1756.

Hansson L, Zanchetti A, Carruthers SG, et al. Effects of intensive blood-pressure lowering and low-dose aspirin in patients with hypertension: principal results of the Hypertension Optimal Treatment (HOT) randomised trial. HOT Study Group. *Lancet.* 1998;351:1755-1762.

Heart Outcomes Prevention Evaluation (HOPE) Study Investigators. Effects of ramipril on cardiovascular and microvascular outcomes in people with diabetes mellitus: results of the HOPE study and MICRO-HOPE substudy. *Lancet.* 2000;355:253-259.

Hypertension Detection and Follow-up Program Cooperative Group. Five-year findings of the hypertension detection and follow-up Program. I. Reduction in mortality in persons with high blood pressure, including mild hypertension. *JAMA.* 1979;242:2562-2571.

Julius S, Weber MA, Kjeldsen SE, et al. The valsartan antihypertensive long-term use evaluation (VALUE) trial: outcomes in patients receiving monotherapy. *Hypertension.* 2006;48:385-391.

Kerr EA, Zikmund-Fisher BJ, Klamerus ML, Subramanian U, Hogan MM, Hofer TP. The role of clinical uncertainty in treatment decisions for diabetic patients with uncontrolled blood pressure. *Ann Intern Med.* 2008;148:717-727.

Lewis EJ, Hunsicker LG, Clarke WR, et al: for the Collaborative Study Group. Renoprotective effect of the angiotensin-receptor anatagonist irbesartan in patients with nephropathy due to type 2 diabetes. *N Engl J Med.* 2001;345:851-860.

Lewis EJ, Hunsicker LG, Bain RP, Rohde RD. The effect of angiotensin-converting-enzyme inhibition on diabetic nephropathy. The Collaborative Study Group [published erratum appears in *N Engl J Med.* 1993;330:152]. *N Engl J Med.* 1993;329:1456-1462.

Lindholm LH, Ibsen H, Dahlof B, et al for the LIFE Study Group. Cardiovascular morbidity and mortality in patients with diabetes in the Losartan Intervention for Endpoint Reduction in Hypertension study (LIFE): a randomised trial against atenolol. *Lancet.* 2002;359:1004-1010.

McInnes GT, Yeo WW, Ramsay L, Moser M. Cardiotoxicity and diuretics: much speculation—little substance. *J Hypertens.* 1992;10:317-335. Editorial.

Moser M. Current hypertension management, separating fact from fiction. *Cleve Clin J Med.* 1993;60:27-37.

Moser M. Is it time for a new approach to the initial treatment of hypertension? *Arch Intern Med.* 2001;161:1040-1045.

Moser M, Hebert PR. Prevention of disease progression, left ventricular hypertrophy and congestive heart failure in the hypertension treatment trials. *J Am Coll Cardiol.* 1996;27:1214-1218.

Multiple Risk Factor Intervention Trial Research Group. Mortality rates after 10.5 years for participants in the Multiple Risk Factor Intervention Trial. Findings related to a priori hypotheses of the trial. *JAMA.* 1990;263:1795-1801.

Parving HH, Lehnert H, Brochner-Mortensen J, Gomis R, Andersen S, Arner P. The effect of irbesartan on the development of diabetic nephropathy in patients with type 2 diabetes. *N Engl J Med.* 2001;345:870-878.

SHEP Investigators. Prevention of stroke by antihypertensive drug treatment in older person with isolated systolic hypertension: final results of the Systolic Hypertension in the Elderly Program (SHEP). *JAMA.* 1991;265:3255-3264.

Sowers JR. Treatment of hypertension in patients with diabetes. *Arch Intern Med.* 2004;164:1850-1857.

Staessen JA, Fagard R, Thijis L, et al for the Systolic Hypertension Europe (Syst-Eur) Trial Investigators. Morbidity and mortality in the placebo-controlled European Trial on Isolated Systolic Hypertension in the Elderly. *Lancet.* 1997;350:757-764.

Tatti P, Pahor M, Byington RP, et al. Outcome results of the Fosinopril Versus Amlodipine Cardiovascular Events Randomized Trial (FACET) in patients with hypertension and NIDDM. *Diabetes Care.* 1998;21:597-603.

United Kingdom Prospective Diabetes Study Group. Tight blood pressure control and risk of macrovascular and microvascular complications in type 2 diabetes: UKPDS 38. UK Prospective Diabetes Study Group. *BMJ.* 1998;317:703-713.

Whelton PK, Barzilay J, Cushman WC, et al; ALLHAT Collaborative Research Group. Clinical outcomes in antihypertensive treatment of type 2 diabetes, impaired fasting glucose concentration, and normoglycemia: Antihypertensive and Lipid-Lowering Treatment to Prevent Heart Attack Trial (ALLHAT). *Arch Intern Med.* 2005;165:1401-1409.

Weir WR, Yeh F, Silverman A, et al. Safety and feasibility of achieving lower systolic blood pressure goals in persons with type 2 diabetes: the SANDS trial. *J Clin Hypertens (Greenwich).* 2009;11:540-548.

7

Hypertension and Diabetes: Cardiovascular Risk Reduction

General Approach

Good BP control has been shown to be an important strategy in reducing both macrovascular and microvascular disease in patients with DM. The target goal for treatment of hypertension in this high-risk population has been set at either 130/85 or 130/80 mm Hg, depending on the organization recommending specific therapy (**Figure 7.1**).

There are a number of unique challenges in adequately treating hypertension in this population. First, many of these patients are overweight and care must be taken in choosing the appropriate-sized cuff so as to avoid errors in BP measurement. Use of a standard-sized BP cuff in an obese patient will often lead to an overestimation of BP levels. This may result in an inappropriate diagnosis of hypertension. A larger sized cuff should be used in such patients.

Second, BP in diabetics is often more labile, especially SBP, than in the general population. This often necessitates more measurements over a longer time period to adequately assess the casual BP. In addition, many persons with diabetes are nondippers and do not experience the normal decrease of about 10% in nocturnal BP. This likely reflects both autonomic dysfunction and/or abnormal renal sensing of supine changes in volume/perfusion pressure (responsiveness of the autonomic nervous system is blunted). This "nondipping" property of BP at night suggests that the office BP measurement may underpredict the 24-hour BP load (**Figure 4.4**). Although ambulatory BP measurements might theoretically be useful in such patients, this is often impractical and probably is unnecessary.

More practical are home BP measurements by the patient. If home BP measurements are to be meaningful, it is important that the validity of the instrument and the technique used by patients in making these measurements

FIGURE 7.1 — Suggested Treatment Program for Patients With Hypertension and Type 2 Diabetes

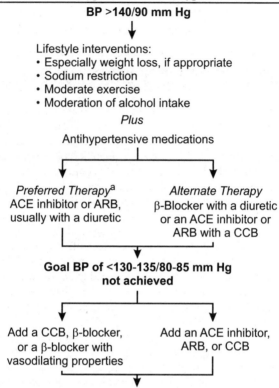

BP >140/90 mm Hg

Lifestyle interventions:
- Especially weight loss, if appropriate
- Sodium restriction
- Moderate exercise
- Moderation of alcohol intake

Plus

Antihypertensive medications

Preferred Therapy[a]
ACE inhibitor or ARB, usually with a diuretic

Alternate Therapy
β-Blocker with a diuretic or an ACE inhibitor or ARB with a CCB

Goal BP of <130-135/80-85 mm Hg not achieved

Add a CCB, β-blocker, or a β-blocker with vasodilating properties

Add an ACE inhibitor, ARB, or CCB

Add one of the drugs not previously given or an α_1-receptor blocker if goal BP is still not achieved

[a] Medications that might be used include an ACE inhibitor (ie, ramipril, accupril, or lisinopril) as monotherapy in dosages from 5 to 20 mg once daily, or in a combination with a diuretic, usually containing 12.5 mg HCTZ. An ARB might be any one listed in **Table 7.9**, ie, losartan (Cozaar) 50 mg titrated up to 100 mg/d, irbesartan (Avapro) 150-300 mg, candesartan (Atacand) 16 mg titrated to 32 mg, or valsartan (Diovan) 80-160 mg, or combinations of these medications, such as Hyzaar (with 12.5 mg of HCTZ), Avalide (with 12.5 mg of HCTZ), Atacand HCT (with 12.5 mg of HCTZ), Diovan HCT (with 12.5 mg of HCTZ), or a combination of an RAAS inhibitor (ACE inhibitor or ARB) and a CCB (ie, amlodipine 5-10 mg).

are monitored. BPs should be measured with a calibrated mercury or aneroid sphygmomanometer on two or three separate office visits to ascertain an appropriate baseline BP unless the first one or two BPs are ≥160/100 mm Hg, in which case a diagnosis of hypertension is justified. Most home BP aneroid or electronic monitors are accurate; finger monitors are probably less so and should be avoided. Because diabetics often are "nondippers," the daytime BP may not reflect the pressure load imposed on the CV system and the kidneys (ie, an office BP of 140/90 mm Hg may be of greater significance in these patients than in nondiabetic subjects whose BPs are lower at night). The failure of BP to decrease at night, especially SBP, may disproportionately increase CVD risk as well as progression of renal disease in diabetic patients. BPs should be measured in the standing position as well as the seated position, especially in the elderly, because diabetics are more likely to have orthostatic decreases in their BP. The standing BP is especially important when titrating therapy.

Utilizing combination therapy should result in goal blood pressure in about 65% to 70% of subjects, whereas monotherapy might only be successful in about 40% to 50% (see *Chapter 6* for a discussion of the *Clinical Uncertainties in Treatment Decisions in Hypertensive Diabetics*).

The Seventh Joint National Committee (JNC 7) on Prevention, Detection, Evaluation, and Treatment of High Blood Pressure has designated BP between 120/80 and 139/89 mm Hg as "prehypertensive." While these levels of BP may not require specific therapy in patients without CV risk factors, some therapy other than lifestyle changes may be required in diabetics.

Essential or primary hypertension is the diagnosis in >90% of diabetic patients with elevated BP. Younger diabetics do not appear to have an increase in secondary forms of hypertension. Because diabetes is more common with increasing age, the physician should be aware of the possibility of renal artery atherosclerosis in these subjects. This condition should also be considered in other elderly patients, especially if the patient has been or is currently a smoker. Obviously, it is important to obtain a serum creatinine, electrolytes, and a spot urine albumin and creatinine for determination of the presence of microalbuminuria. It should be remembered that renal parenchymal disease, which occurs in approximately 20% of patients with type 2 diabetes and in one third of people with type 1 diabetes, is an important predictor of progression of hypertension in these patients. The presence of microalbuminuria indicates greater risk for a MI and stroke as well as the progression of renal disease. Therefore, the presence of microalbuminuria necessitates more rigorous control of BP and other CV risk factors as indicated in the guidelines from JNC 7 and from the ADA. The presence of a creatinine level of >1.5 mg/dL is also an indication for more aggressive therapy. BP levels of 120/75 mm Hg would be an appropriate therapeutic target in such patients. This may not always be achieved, but attempts to lower BP to these levels should be made.

Therapy in patients with hypertension and diabetes should include lifestyle modifications, especially involving weight reduction, increased aerobic activity, and moderation of salt and alcohol intake (**Table 7.1**). Most experts believe that medications should be started at the same time as lifestyle interventions in these patients since diabetics, even with stage or grade 1 hypertension, are in a high-risk category (**Table 7.2**). Most diabetics with definite elevations of BP will require medication to achieve goal BP. Based on previously described clinical trial results, ACE inhibitors, low-dose diuretics, CCBs, ARBs, and in some cases β-blockers may be initial medication choices (depending on the presence or absence of other comorbidities, ie, in patients with angina or post MI, a β-blocker might be selected; in other instances, it might be a third or fourth choice). As noted, most hypertensive diabetic patients will need more than one agent; a diuretic is usually needed to achieve the therapeutic BP goal of 130/80-85 mm Hg. For that reason, JNC 7 suggests the use of the two medications as appropriate initial therapy in diabetic hypertensives, especially in patients with BP >160/100 mm Hg.

TABLE 7.1 — Lifestyle Modifications for Control of Hypertension

- Weight loss, if overweight[a]
- Reduction of sodium intake to <100 mmol/d (2.4 g sodium or approximately 6 g sodium chloride)[a]
- Limit alcohol intake to <1 oz/d of ethanol (24 oz beer, 10 oz wine, or 2 oz 80-proof whiskey); approximately one half of these amounts for women and thin people
- Cessation of smoking and reduction of dietary saturated fat and cholesterol for overall CV health; reduced fat intake also helps reduce caloric intake—important for control of weight and type 2 diabetes
- Maintain adequate dietary potassium, calcium, and magnesium intake
- Relaxation techniques—biofeedback
- Vegetarian diets, fish oil

[a] These interventions have been found to be most effective. Data on other interventions are not definitive (see text).

Modified from: The JNC 7 Report. *JAMA*. 2003;289:2560-2572.

7

Nonpharmacologic Treatment

The first approach to the treatment of hypertension in diabetics, as well as in nondiabetics, should be lifestyle modifications. Estimates of how much BP might be lowered by lifestyle changes (if they are carefully adhered to) are listed in **Table 7.3**. In some cases, this degree of BP change will represent adequate treatment, but most patients with hypertension will require medication to achieve goal BP.

Initial efforts should include weight loss, if appropriate. Weight reduction is probably the single most important nondrug intervention. This may be especially important in diabetic subjects. Obesity is present in >60% of diabetics and hyperlipidemia is also a common finding. Losing weight and reducing lipid levels should be a major priority. But most people are unaware of their so-called ideal weight and when they are told to lose weight, they do not have a good idea of a goal or ideal weight. Of course, looking in a mirror will often help to determine whether someone is overweight, but there are more scientific and quite simple ways to do this.

TABLE 7.2 — Risk Stratification of Hypertension to Guide Treatment Choices[a,b]

BP Stage (mm Hg)	Initial Therapy[c]		
	Risk Group A No risk factors; no TOD/CVD	Risk Group B At least one risk factor, not including diabetes	Risk Group C TOD or evidence of CVD and/or diabetes, with/without no TOD/CV other risk factors
130-139/85-89	Lifestyle modification	Lifestyle modification	Medication
140-159/90-99 (stage 1)	Lifestyle modification (2-3 months)	Lifestyle modification[d] (2-4 weeks)	Medication
≥160/≥100 (stage 2)	Medication	Medication	Medication

[a] Modified from JNC-VI and JNC 7.

[b] Lifestyle modification should be adjunctive therapy for all patients recommended for pharmacologic therapy.

[c] For example, a patient with diabetes and a BP of 142/94 mm Hg plus LVH should be classified as having stage 1 hypertension with TOD (LVH) and with another major risk factor (diabetes). Patient would be stage 1, risk group C; pharmacologic treatment should be initiated at the same time as lifestyle modifications.

[d] For patients with multiple risk factors, clinicians should consider drugs plus lifestyle modifications as initial therapy.

TABLE 7.3 — Lifestyle Modifications

	Approximate SBP Reduction (Range/mm Hg)
Weight reduction	5-20/10 kg of weight loss
DASH eating plan	8-14
Dietary sodium reduction	2-8
Physical activity	4-9
Moderation of alcohol consumption	2-4

The JNC 7 Report. *JAMA*. 2003;289:2560-2572.

Although BMI is used by many physicians to define overweight or obesity and target BMIs are set for patients, this is often confusing. **Table 7.4** outlines how to calculate the BMI and defines the limits of normal. A more simple method that is reasonably accurate in calculating ideal weight is noted in **Table 7.5**. These numbers are not set in granite and a variance of 5 to 10 lb is reasonable.

The next question is, How many calories does a patient need to maintain weight or lose weight? Again, a simple formula is helpful (**Table 7.6**). With these

7

TABLE 7.4 — Calculating Body Mass Index and Desirable Ranges

BMI = Weight (kg) ÷ Height (meters) Squared

To convert pounds to kilograms, divide by 2.2:
$$220\text{-lb} \div 2.2 = 100 \text{ kg}$$

To convert height in inches to meters, divide by 39.4:
$$74 \text{ inches} \div 39.4 = 1.9 \text{ meters [squared} = 3.6]$$

Calculating the BMI of a person 1.9 meters tall and weighing 100 kg:
$$100 \text{ kg} \div 3.6 = \text{BMI of } 28$$

	BMI	
	Men	Women
Desirable range	22-24	21-23
Overweight	>28	>27
Seriously overweight	>32-33	>31

TABLE 7.5 — Simple Method of Calculating Ideal Weight[a]

Women

  100 lb for first 5 ft of height
  Add 5 lb for each additional inch of height
  Example: 5′ 5″ woman = $100 + (5 \times 5) = 125$ lb

Men

  106 lb for first 5 ft of height
  Add 6 lb for each additional inch of height
  Example: 6′ man = $106 + (12 \times 6) = 178$ lb

[a] Plus or minus 5 to 10 lb.

TABLE 7.6 — Calculating Calories to Maintain or Lose Weight

Calculating Daily Caloric Intake Necessary to Maintain Ideal Body Weight

Ideal weight × Level of physical activity

Example: maintaining ideal weight of 125 lb:

Sedentary	13	$125 \times 13 = 1625$ calories/d
Moderately active	15	$125 \times 15 = 1875$ calories/d
Active	17	$125 \times 17 = 2125$ calories/d

Calculating Daily Caloric Intake Reduction Necessary to Lose Weight

Reducing caloric intake by 500 calories/d will result in weight loss of 1 lb/wk ($500 \times 7 = 3500$ calories/wk), or reduce intake by 300 calories/d and exercise to burn 200 calories/d.

Example: If a moderately active individual can maintain body weight with 1875 calories/d, a 500-calories/d reduction over 1 week will be necessary to lose 1 lb of body weight ($1875 - 500 = 1375$ calories/d × 7 days).

guidelines, the patient and physician may embark on a reasonable diet program. Even a 10-lb weight loss may result in a decrease in BP so that specific medication may not be necessary. Weight loss will also frequently help to reduce lipid levels and will increase insulin sensitivity and help to control blood glucose levels.

While maintaining an ideal weight or losing weight is an appropriate first step in all hypertensive individuals, it is especially important in diabetics. A low-calorie, low–saturated-fat diet should therefore be advised. Data also indicate that maintaining appropriate weight or losing weight may actually prevent the development of hypertension. Diabetic patients should consult their physicians before going on one of the popular low-carbohydrate or high-protein, high-fat diets. To reemphasize, people may lose weight while on these diets but there are very few data on their long-term effects. There are abundant data, for example, to suggest that people on a high-fat diet are at increased risk for heart disease. It should be remembered that most diabetic hypertensive individuals will require one or more antihypertensive drugs in addition to weight loss or other lifestyle changes to lower their BP to goal levels.

A decrease in sodium (salt) intake is also indicated despite ongoing controversies about the benefits of salt restriction. Data link a high salt intake to elevated BP and a lower intake to some reduction in BP. Diabetics appear to be salt sensitive; BP responds to salt restriction to a greater degree in these individuals than in many other hypertensive subjects, especially if they are >60 years of age. Therefore, limitation of sodium intake is especially important in diabetics if they have hypertension (BP >140/90 mm Hg or even lower BP of 130-135/80-85 mm Hg). Restriction need not be severe; most patients will not tolerate a very–low-sodium diet for long periods of time. A limited intake of heavily salted foods—pretzels, salted peanuts, hot dogs, processed meats, canned soups, etc—and limitation of salt in cooking and at the table will probably reduce intake to the presently recommended 6 g of salt (2.4 g sodium) per day. A good rule in selecting prepared foods is to avoid (if possible) foods with a sodium content of >150 mg per serving—*read labels*. **Table 7.7** lists foods to be avoided or markedly limited (see *Chapter 10* for a review of lifestyle changes that should be made in all diabetics).

Data suggest that further limitations to 1.5 g of sodium per day will reduce BP to a greater degree. This level of restricted intake is more difficult to achieve because of the amount of processed food that people consume, but it might be possible without a drastic

TABLE 7.7 — Some High-Sodium–Content Foods That Should Be Avoided

• Potato chips	• Bouillon
• Pretzels	• Ham
• Salted crackers	• Sausages
• Biscuits	• Frankfurters
• Pancakes	• Smoked meats or fish
• Fast foods	• Sardines
• Olives	• Tomato juice (canned)
• Pickles	• Frozen lima beans
• Sauerkraut	• Frozen peas
• Soy sauce	• Canned spinach
• Catsup	• Canned carrots
• Many kinds of cheese	
• Commercially prepared soups or stews	
• Pastries or cakes made from self-rising flour mixes	

modification of diet. The Dietary Approaches to Stop Hypertension (DASH) diet, which is a balanced diet consisting of fruits, vegetables, and low-fat dairy products along with a low sodium content, is a reasonable diet for hypertensive diabetics to follow.

As repeatedly noted, the JNC 7 has suggested BP levels <140/90 mm Hg as a goal for nondiabetic individuals, but levels of <130/80-85 mm Hg for diabetic patients. Evidence indicates that lower BP levels in diabetic hypertensives reduce CV events to a greater degree. Increasing evidence from clinical trials has led to the recommendations of a committee of the National Kidney Foundation and the ADA that BP goals in the diabetic should be <130/80-85 mm Hg or *as low as possible consistent with treatment that does not cause annoying symptoms.*

Pharmacologic Therapy

Once the decision is made to treat a hypertensive diabetic patient with medication, a choice of initial therapy must be made. Diabetic hypertensives fall into the high-risk category, and the JNC 7, as well as other national committees, has recommended that medication be started initially at the same time as lifestyle changes.

Medication should be started at the same time as weight loss, a low-sodium diet, and an exercise program.

Some physicians still believe that a trial of nonpharmacologic interventions alone is justified for a period of time ranging from 1 to 3 months, depending on the level of BP, but we agree with the JNC 7 approach. In addition, as noted, many of these individuals will not respond to goal levels of BP with one medication. It is therefore recommended by the JNC 7 committee that multiple agents (alone or in combination) can be given as initial therapy. Among the medications that have proven effective in reducing BP as well as morbidity/mortality in diabetic hypertensives are the ACE inhibitors, diuretics, ARBs, and β-blockers. Data on the CCBs are less definitive except in the elderly. These medications will reduce BP and reduce the occurrence of stroke, but some studies suggest that they may not be as effective as an ACE inhibitor plus a diuretic in reducing CHD events, progression of renal disease in diabetics, and especially heart failure.

A recent study, however, reports that an overall reduction of 20% of CV events was noted in patients who received an ACE inhibitor/CCB regimen compared with those who were on an ACE inhibitor/diuretic regimen. About 60% of the patients in the Avoiding Cardiovascular Events Through Combination Therapy in Patients Living With Systolic Hypertension (ACCOMPLISH) study were diabetics. Outcome benefits were similar in these subjects and the nondiabetic subjects. Use of an ACE inhibitor/ CCB combination compared with an ACE inhibitor/ diuretic resulted in an absolute reduction of composite CV events and death from CV events of 2.2% (8.8% compared with 11%) in diabetic patients. Differences were significant (**Table 7.8**).

It is of interest that while baseline characteristics and CV risk factors were similar in the two treatment groups, events were actually higher in nondiabetics than in diabetics. This is difficult to explain in view of extensive data indicating a higher CV morbidity and mortality in diabetics compared to patients with normoglycemia.

In ALLHAT, which included 14,000 diabetic patients, there was no difference in primary CHD out-

TABLE 7.8 — ACCOMPLISH Trial: Composite of CV Events and Deaths From CVD

	Benazepril/ CCB (%)	Benazepril/ HCTZ (%)	Absolute Difference (%)
Age			
>65 yo	10.1	12.4	2.3
>70 yo	11.0	13.8	2.8
Diabetes			
Yes	8.8	11.0	2.2
No	10.8	12.9	2.1

Jamerson K, et al. *N Engl J Med.* 2008;359:2417-2428.

come (fatal and nonfatal MIs) among the three agents tested (eg, ACE inhibitor, dihydropyridine CCB, and diuretic). There were, however, fewer cases of heart failure with the diuretic compared with the CCB.

Some trials report that CHD morbidity and mortality rates in hypertensive nondiabetics and hypertensive diabetics are not significantly different when a CCB is used as baseline therapy when compared with rates in patients treated with an ARB or ACE inhibitor. However, there are data from other smaller trials (FACET, ABCD trial, African American Study of Kidney Disease and Hypertension trial, etc) that cannot be discounted and suggest a benefit of RAAS inhibitors compared with CCB therapy in diabetic patients, especially those with nephropathy and proteinuria.

New-Onset Diabetes With Antihypertensive Medications

In the 5-year ALLHAT trial, 9.8% of the CCB-treated patients developed NOD compared with 11.6% in the diuretic group and 8.1% in the ACE inhibitor group. The difference between the ACE inhibitor and diuretic groups was significant—the ACE inhibitor/CCB difference was 1.8% and not significant.

The VALUE trial that evaluated an ARB-treated and a CCB-treated group of high-risk subjects also reported fewer NOD cases in the ARB group than in the CCB group (13.1% compared with 16.4%; $P = 0.0001$).

As is evident from the previous discussion, there are some differences in the occurrence of NOD between different classes of medications. The clinical significance of these changes has been questioned. As noted, some data from the SHEP and ALLHAT trials indicate that the occurrence of NOD does not influence long-term CVD outcome. It should be reemphasized that hypertensive patients are more prone to develop diabetes than nonhypertensive patients, regardless of specific treatment.

Newer data from the ALLHAT trial regarding results in normoglycemic and diabetic patients, as well as in patients with IFG, appear to indicate that a diuretic-based treatment (often with a β-blocker added) is as or more effective in controlling CHD, combined CV events, heart failure, and strokes as therapy based on an ACE inhibitor (lisinopril) or a CCB (amlodipine). In addition, the occurrence of ESRD does not differ between the ACE inhibitor– and diuretic-based regimens (**Figure 7.2** and **Figure 7.3**).

There is no question that intensive BP control reduces mortality/morbidity in diabetic patients regardless of the medication used. Until we have more consistent or definitive data on the clinical significance of NOD, it should not be a primary concern when choosing a medication for initial therapy. However, in certain high-risk patients, the use of an RAAS blocker may be the initial drug of choice.

A suggested treatment program for patients with hypertension and type 2 diabetes is presented in **Figure 7.1**.

■ Angiotensin-Converting Enzyme Inhibitors

ACE inhibitors have been recommended as initial antihypertensive therapy in diabetic persons with proteinuria. These medications usually must be given with a diuretic to gain better BP control. They have been shown to protect against deterioration due to renal disease (diabetic nephropathy) as well as progression of proteinuria. These effects of ACE inhibitors have been observed in normotensive as well as hypertensive patients with diabetes. As repeatedly emphasized, it is now recognized that proteinuria is a predictor of CVD as well as diabetic nephropathy.

FIGURE 7.2 — ALLHAT: Hazard Ratios and Relative Risks With a CCB (Amlodipine) Compared With Chlorthalidone in Normoglycemic Patients, Diabetic Patients, and Those With Impaired Fasting Glucose Levels

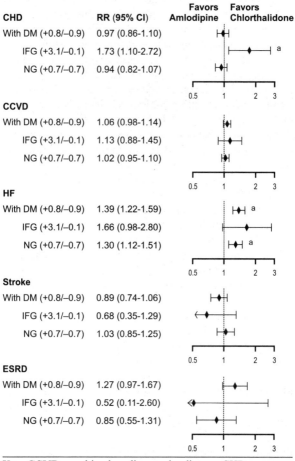

CHD	RR (95% CI)
With DM (+0.8/–0.9)	0.97 (0.86-1.10)
IFG (+3.1/–0.1)	1.73 (1.10-2.72) [a]
NG (+0.7/–0.7)	0.94 (0.82-1.07)

CCVD	RR (95% CI)
With DM (+0.8/–0.9)	1.06 (0.98-1.14)
IFG (+3.1/–0.1)	1.13 (0.88-1.45)
NG (+0.7/–0.7)	1.02 (0.95-1.10)

HF	RR (95% CI)
With DM (+0.8/–0.9)	1.39 (1.22-1.59) [a]
IFG (+3.1/–0.1)	1.66 (0.98-2.80)
NG (+0.7/–0.7)	1.30 (1.12-1.51) [a]

Stroke	RR (95% CI)
With DM (+0.8/–0.9)	0.89 (0.74-1.06)
IFG (+3.1/–0.1)	0.68 (0.35-1.29)
NG (+0.7/–0.7)	1.03 (0.85-1.25)

ESRD	RR (95% CI)
With DM (+0.8/–0.9)	1.27 (0.97-1.67)
IFG (+3.1/–0.1)	0.52 (0.11-2.60)
NG (+0.7/–0.7)	0.85 (0.55-1.31)

Key: CCVD, combined cardiovascular disease; CHD, coronary heart disease; DM, diabetes mellitus; ESRD, end-stage renal disease; HF, heart failure; NG, normoglycemic.

No evidence to suggest that outcome was improved in the CCB group compared with the diuretic-based treatment group.

[a] Statistically significant difference.

Adapted from: Wright JT Jr, et al. *Arch Intern Med*. 2009;169:832-842.

FIGURE 7.3 — ALLHAT: Clinical Outcomes for an Angiotensin-Converting Enzyme Inhibitor Compared With Chlorthalidone[a] in Prespecified Subgroups

CHD	RR (95% CI)	Favors Lisinopril / Favors Chlorthalidone
With DM (+2.2/–0.1)	0.97 (0.85-1.10)	
IFG (+2.0/–0.2)	1.16 (0.71-1.89)	
NG (+1.2/+0.3)	1.02 (0.89-1.16)	
CCVD		
With DM (+2.2/–0.1)	1.07 (0.99-1.15)	
IFG (+2.0/–0.2)	1.09 (0.85-1.39)	
NG (+1.2/+0.3)	1.13 (1.05-1.22)	[b]
HF		
With DM (+2.2/–0.1)	1.15 (1.00-1.32)	
IFG (+2.0/–0.2)	1.20 (0.69-2.09)	
NG (+1.2/+0.3)	1.19 (1.02-1.39)	[b]
Stroke		
With DM (+2.2/–0.1)	1.06 (0.89-1.26)	
IFG (+2.0/–0.2)	0.91 (0.52-1.61)	
NG (+1.2/+0.3)	1.31 (1.10-1.57)	[b]
ESRD		
With DM (+2.2/–0.1)	1.09 (0.82-1.46)	
IFG (+2.0/–0.2)	1.50 (0.48-4.66)	
NG (+1.2/+0.3)	0.99 (0.65-1.50)	

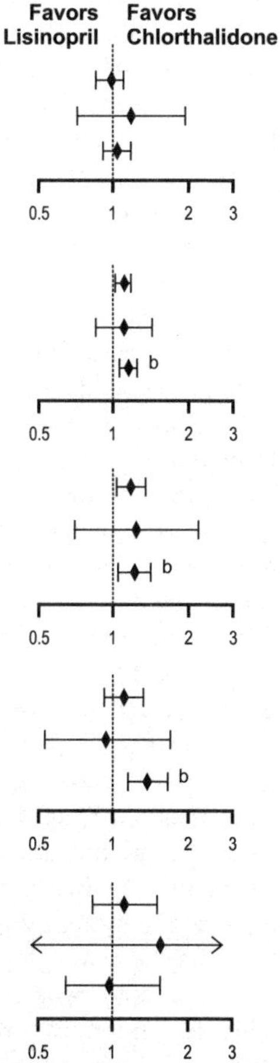

Key: CCVD, combined cardiovascular disease; CHD, coronary heart disease; DM, diabetes mellitus; ESRD, end-stage renal disease; HF, heart failure; NG, normoglycemic.

No evidence that ACE inhibitor results were better than diuretic-based treatment in diabetic patients with IFG or normoglycemic levels.

[a] 12.5 to 25 mg/d.
[b] Statistically significant difference.

Adapted from: Wright JT Jr, et al. *Arch Intern Med.* 2009;169:832-842.

It is not surprising therefore that ACE inhibitor therapy has resulted in reductions in MI and stroke. As previously noted, a cardioprotective effect of ACE inhibitors over and above that which may be provided by CCBs in diabetic patients was suggested by the results of the smaller ABCD and FACET studies. In addition, the CAPPP and the HOPE trials also demonstrated a reduction of CV events in diabetics with the use of an ACE inhibitor. The results of the HOPE and CAPPP trials indicate that the use of ACE inhibitors when added to other medications not only reduces macrovascular and microvascular disease in diabetic hypertensive patients but also may prevent the development of type 2 diabetes in some hypertensive patients. This finding might have been anticipated since, as noted, these patients are often insulin-resistant and have a 2- to 3-fold greater propensity to develop type 2 diabetes than normotensive persons. ACE inhibitor–induced improvement of insulin resistance may be explained by improved blood flow to the skeletal muscle microcirculation as well as improved insulin action at the tissue level. **Table 7.9** lists information about the available ACE inhibitors.

■ **Angiotensin Receptor Blockers**

Clinical trial data also support the role of ARBs in high-risk patients, such as those with diabetes and hypertension. These agents may prove effective in some cases that are not controlled with ACE inhibition. This is based on a number of factors. First, inhibition of converting enzyme by ACE inhibitors may not be sustained over time, as these agents are competitive inhibitors whose blockade may be overridden by increased angiotensin I levels. This may result from increased renin production as a result of the loss of feedback inhibition. In an unblocked renin system, the generation of angiotensin II tends to suppress renin production. If angiotensin II is not generated as a result of ACE inhibition, this feedback loop is interrupted, more renin is generated, and more angiotensin I is produced; this may overwhelm ACE blockade with some production of angiotensin II. Further, there is increasing evidence that alternative pathways of conversion of angiotensin I to angiotensin II may restore

TABLE 7.9 — ACE Inhibitors Used for Treating Hypertension

Generic (Trade) Name	Usual Dosage Range (mg)	Frequency	Adverse Reactions	Physiologic Effects	Comments
Benazepril (Lotensin)	10-40	1 or 2/d	*Cough*, rash, loss of taste, palpitations, rarely angio-edema	Blocks formation of angiotensin II, promoting vasodilation and decreased aldosterone; also increases bradykinin and vasodilator prostaglandins	• Diuretic doses should be reduced before starting ACE inhibitor whenever possible to prevent excessive hypotension
Captopril (Capoten)	25-150	2 or 3/d			• Smaller doses in patients with serum creatinine >3 mg/dL
Enalapril (Vasotec)	2.5-40	1 or 2/d			• May cause hyperkalemia in patients with renal impairment or in those receiving postassium-sparing agents
Fosinopril (Monopril)	10-40	1/d			• Can cause renal failure in patients with bilateral renal artery stenosis
Lisinopril (Zestril, Prinivil)	10-40	1/d			
Moexipril (Univasc)	7.5-30	1 or 2/d			
Perindopril (Aceon)	4-8	1 or 2/d			
Quinapril (Accupril)	10-80	1 or 2/d			
Ramipril (Altace)	2.5-20	1 or 2/d			
Trandolapril (Mavik)	1-4	1/d			

7

153

circulating or tissue levels of angiotensin II despite ACE inhibition. Indeed, circulating angiotensin II levels may return toward pretreatment levels during long-term ACE inhibitor therapy.

ARBs competitively block the AT_1 receptor subtype in peripheral tissues. The AT_1 receptor mediates the known CV and renal effects of angiotensin II. Studies in animal models of diabetic renal disease have shown that ARBs, like ACE inhibitors, reduce the progression of microalbuminuria and renal dysfunction. One study in patients with diabetic renal disease confirmed that valsartan and the ACE inhibitor captopril are equally effective in decreasing urinary protein excretion. Trials with losartan and irbesartan confirm the beneficial effects of these agents in patients with either microproteinuria or >300 mg/day of proteinuria or with elevated creatinine levels. The ONTARGET results also indicate that an ARB is as effective in reducing CV events as an ACE inhibitor.

Diabetic patients with cardiomyopathy may also benefit from using an ACE inhibitor and ARB together. In the Randomized Evaluation of Strategies for Left Ventricular Dysfunction (RESOLV) trial, the combination of the ARB candesartan and the ACE inhibitor enalapril was well tolerated, but the study was not powered to evaluate effects on long-term outcome comparing the ARB or ACE inhibitor alone. Additional studies have evaluated the impact of combinations of ARB and ACE inhibitor therapy on renal disease and CVD as well as on mortality in diabetic patients with hypertension. It does not appear that the combination of an ACE inhibitor or ARB will reduce CV events to a greater degree than an ACE inhibitor–based regimen alone.

ARBs are listed in JNC 7 as one of the initial therapies for hypertension in diabetic patients, and based on trial data, the ADA has recommended these agents as a preferred first-step drug in these patients. The RENAAL, IDNT, and IRMA 2 trial results all indicated that a program based on ARB therapy compared with a program not including an ARB will reduce the progression of renal disease from less severe to more severe and will reduce the progression to ESRD in type 2 hypertensive diabetics with proteinuria.

The ability of the ARBs to reduce proteinuria suggests that these blocking agents may also protect against CVD. Trials with these agents, such as the LIFE study, provide us with indications about the use of these drugs in reducing CVD in diabetic patients. The ARBs can be used instead of ACE inhibitors in diabetic patients, in part because they are well tolerated without the occurrence of a cough and considerably less risk of angioedema. Data suggest that an ARB-based treatment program provides comparable CVD risk reduction over time in this high-risk group of patients. **Table 7.10** lists available ARBs.

The VALUE study was designed to answer the question as to whether the use of a regimen based on an ARB (valsartan 80-160 mg/day) would result in a better outcome than a regimen based on a CCB (amlodipine 5-10 mg/day) in a high-risk group of 15,245 patients (46% with evidence of CHD). Hydrochlorothiazide was added to help achieve goal BP. At the end of >4 years, there was no difference between groups in overall cardiac end points but some difference in specific events, ie, MIs were significantly lower (25.8%) in the CCB group.

Sixty-four percent of the CCB group and 58% of the ARB subjects achieved SBP <140 mm Hg. There was a difference in BP levels, especially at 1 month and 6 months (–4/–2 mm Hg and –2.1/–1.6 mm Hg) with the CCB. In the opinion of the investigators, this was consistent with the outcome and further evidence that BP lowering, especially in the early months, makes a difference. However, when groups of patients with an equivalent decrease in BP were compared, there were no differences in outcome between the CCB and the ARB groups. As noted, a definite finding in the VALUE trial was the occurrence of fewer cases of NOD in the ARB group compared with the CCB patients.

■ Diuretics

Thiazide diuretics in relatively low doses (equivalent to about 25 mg/day hydrochlorothiazide or about 15 mg/day chlorthalidone) are effective and safe antihypertensive agents in type 2 diabetic patients. In the SHEP study, adults with type 2 diabetes derived at least as much benefit in stroke and coronary heart disease reduction as

TABLE 7.10 — Angiotensin II Receptor Blockers Used for Treating Hypertension

Generic (Trade) Name	Usual Dosage Range (mg)	Frequency	Adverse Reactions	Physiologic Effects	Comments
Candesartan cilexetil (Atacand)	8-32	1 or 2/d	Occasional dizziness; generally well tolerated	Blocks action of angiotensin II; → vasodilation; ↓ aldosterone secretion	• Whenever possible, diuretic doses should be reduced before starting ARBs to prevent excessive hypotension
Eprosartan mesylate (Teveten)	400-800	1 or 2/d			• Reduce dose in patients with serum creatinine >3.0 md/dL
Irbesartan (Avapro)	150-300	1/d			• Can cause renal failure in patients with bilateral renal artery stenosis
Losartan potassium (Cozaar)	25-100	1 or 2/d			
Olmesartan medoxomil (Benicar)	20-40	1/d			
Telmisartan (Micardis)	20-80	1/d			
Valsartan (Diovan)	80-320	1/d			

those without diabetes. Diuretics in relatively low doses are not generally associated with metabolic abnormalities.

The use of a diuretic or diuretic/β-blocker–based regimen in several large trials (ie, STOP-2, UKPDS) reduced morbidity/mortality and lowered BP to a degree equal to other antihypertensive agents in hypertensive diabetic subjects. These agents are often a necessary part of the antihypertensive regimen in diabetic patients because they are often salt sensitive and have expanded plasma volumes. A majority of diabetic patients will not achieve goal BPs of <130-135/80-85 mm Hg without the use of a diuretic. Some experts believe that chlorthalidone in low doses may be the diuretic of choice because of its long duration of activity.

Information about available thiazide diuretics is listed in **Table 7.11**. Concerns about possible adverse effects of these agents on glucose metabolism are addressed in *Chapter 5*.

■ β-Blockers

β-Blockers are useful agents in the treatment of hypertension in diabetic patients, especially those who are post MI or have angina or heart failure. For many years, physicians were advised not to use these medications in diabetics or to use them with care. Clinical trials, however, have confirmed that β-blockers are safe and effective in diabetic patients. In the UKPDS, an atenolol-based treatment program reduced microvascular complications of diabetes by 37%, stroke by 44%, and death related to diabetes by 32% in patients whose BP was lowered to a greater degree than patients who achieved higher levels of BP. The atenolol regimen was equally as effective as a captopril-based program in reducing microvascular and macrovascular complications of diabetes (as discussed before, BP control—not a specific medication—appeared to make the difference in outcome). The ability of β-blockers to suppress the renin-angiotensin system may, in part, account for this beneficial result. As noted, β-Blockers are especially indicated in diabetic patients with known coronary artery disease.

Generally, there are no major problems with β-blockers with regard to worsening hyperglycemic

7

TABLE 7.11 — Some Commonly Used Diuretics for Treating Hypertension

Generic (Trade) Name	Usual Dosage Range (mg)	Frequency	Duration of Action (h)	Comments
Chlorthalidone (Hygroton, Thalitone)	12.5-25	1/d	24-72	More effective than loop diuretics except in patient with serum creatinine >2.5 mg/dL— hydrochlorothiazide or chlorthalidone was used in most clinical trials
	15	1/d	24-72	
Hydrochlorothiazide (Hydrodiuril, Microzide)	12.5-50	1-2/d	12-18	
Indapamide (Lozol)	1.25-5.0	1/d	18-24	A relatively low-sodium and high-potassium diet may help to augment BP lowering and prevent hypokalemia
Methyclothiazide (Enduron)	2.5-5	1/d	>24	
Metolazone (Mykrox, Zaroxolyn)	0.5-5	1/d	18-24	

control or in causing or masking hypoglycemia in most patients with type 2 diabetes. The use of carvedilol, a β-blocker with vasodilating properties, has less effect on glucose metabolism than a β-blocker without α-blocking properties. Carvedilol has antioxidant and antiproliferative properties, is an effective BP-lowering agent, and does not increase vascular resistance. Nebivolol, a β-blocker with antioxidant and vasodilatory properties (the result of nitric oxide enhancement) has also been shown to have less effect on glucose metabolism than a β-blocker without vasodilatory properties. This agent has also been found to be effective in the treatment of heart failure in the elderly.

Some reports suggest an increase in the risk of developing hyperglycemia with the use of either a β-blocker or a diuretic, but this was not noted when antihypertensive agents were compared in one review of data in treated patients (**Figure 7.4**). As noted, while hypertensive individuals are at greater risk for developing diabetes than nonhypertensives regardless of treatment, there was no difference in risk associated with different medications. In a prospective study of >12,000 patients, however, after adjustments for age, gender, activity level, family history, adiposity, etc, a 28% increase in NOD was found in patients taking a β-blocker compared with those not on any medication. In this study, risk was not increased in patients on a diuretic, ACE inhibitor, or CCB. The authors stated that "concern about this risk of diabetes should not discourage physicians from prescribing thiazide diuretics to nondiabetic adults who have hypertension. The use of β-blockers appears to increase the risk of diabetes, but this adverse effect must be weighed against the proven benefits of β-blockers in reducing the risk of CV events."

A randomized double-blind study, Glycemic Effects in Diabetic Mellitus: Carvedilol-Metoprolol Comparison in Hypertensives (GEMINI), evaluated 1235 type 2 diabetics with a mean age of 61 years. A 5-month maintenance period compared the use of metoprolol (average dose 128 mg bid) with carvedilol (average dose 17.5 mg bid) when added to baseline therapy of an ACE inhibitor or an ARB (**Table 7.12**). Baseline BPs were 149/86 mm

FIGURE 7.4 — Risk of Hyperglycemia With Use of Antihypertensive Drugs

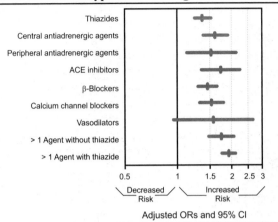

Risk for development of hyperglycemia requiring treatment with antidiabetic drugs in users of antihypertensive drugs relative to nonusers. Note increased risk overall in hypertensive subjects compared with nonhypertensives, but no difference between drugs.

Gutwitz HJ, et al. *Ann Intern Med.* 1993;118:273-278.

Hg and 149/87 mm Hg, respectively. More than 40% of patients required the addition of hydrochlorothiazide and >20% required a CCB to control BP. No BP or plasma glucose level differences were noted between the two groups. However, patients experienced statistically significantly more of an increase in HbA_{1C} with metoprolol (0.15%) than with carvedilol (0.02%)—a difference of 0.13%. Twice as many patients on metoprolol noted an increase in HbA_{1C} of 1.0%. The carvedilol group experienced an increase in insulin sensitivity, less progression to microalbuminuria, and significantly less of an increase in serum triglyceride levels.

This study confirms both the need for multiple medications to reduce BPs to goal levels in diabetic patients (even in people with less severe hypertension) and that a β-blocker with α-blocking capabilities may be preferred in diabetic patients because of its beneficial effect on glycemic control, insulin sensitivity, and some

TABLE 7.12 — GEMINI Study: Comparison of Carvedilol and Metoprolol in Diabetic Patients[a]

Study Outcome Measures	Carvedilol (n=454)		Metoprolol (n=657)		P Value[b]
	Baseline	35 Weeks	Baseline	35 Weeks	
Mean BP (mm Hg)	149/87	131/77	149/86	132/77	NS
Plasma glucose (mg/dL)	147	155	147	157	NS
Mean albumin/creatinine ratio	13	11	12	13	0.003
Triglycerides	159	168	168	186	<0.001
HbA$_{1C}$	**7.2**	**7.22**	**7.2**	**7.35**	**0.004**

[a] A study of 1235 patients aged 35 to 86 years with type 2 diabetes and hypertension who were also receiving an ACE inhibitor or an ARB; >40% received hydrochlorothiazide and 25% received CCBs in order to achieve BP target.
[b] Carvedilol compared with metoprolol.

Bakris GL, et al. *JAMA*. 2004;292:2227-2236.

7

of the manifestations of the metabolic syndrome, which are frequently noted in type 2 diabetics.

A meta-analysis of results from trials utilizing β-blockers as initial therapy compared with other antihypertensive drugs suggests that stroke is reduced to a lesser degree with β-blockers. On the basis of these data, some investigators and guidelines suggest that β-blockers should no longer be considered as initial therapy or even Step 2 or 3 therapy except in patients with angina or CHD. This recommendation may not apply, however, to β-blockers with vasodilatory properties. At present, there are no long-term CVD outcome studies available with these agents.

Some concerns still exist, however, that β-blockers may cause hypoglycemia and mask symptoms of hypoglycemia in patients with type 1 diabetes and in type 2 diabetics with severe autonomic neuropathy. Available β-blockers and their dosing information are listed in **Table 7.13**.

■ **Calcium Channel Blockers**

CCBs are often useful in conjunction with other drugs, particularly if diuretics, ACE inhibitors, or ARBs, alone or in combination, are not effective in controlling the BP of a diabetic hypertensive. These agents were the initial therapeutic agents in SYST-EUR and the HOT study. In both of these trials, diabetic persons had a significantly greater reduction in CVD events than did the nondiabetic hypertensive cohort. Most of these patients, as in all the other trials, required several medications to reach the more optimal SBP and DBP levels.

Some current recommendations suggest that CCBs are not the preferred medications for initial antihypertensive therapy, but should be considered as add-on or substitute therapy in those diabetics who cannot be controlled or cannot tolerate ACE inhibitors, ARBs, and/ or diuretics. These agents are generally metabolically neutral. As noted, the VALUE and ASCOT studies suggest that a long-acting dihydropyridine CCB is as effective as the comparator agents in reducing BP and overall CHD events. As also noted, those medications may not be as effective in diabetic nephropathy or in preventing congestive heart failure. In ALLHAT, the occurrence of CHF was greater with a CCB than with a diuretic-based regimen. Short-acting dihydropyridine CCBs should not be and are no longer used in diabetic patients because of the potential of increased CVD events in this high-risk population.

Recent data suggest that an ACE inhibitor/CCB-based regimen is effective in reducing CV events to a greater degree than an ACE inhibitor/diuretic–treatment program.

■ Renin Inhibitors

Renin, which is secreted by the kidney in response to decreases in blood volume and renal perfusion, cleaves angiotensinogen to angiotensin I, thereby contributing to the cascade leading to increased levels of angiotensin II. Thus inhibition of renin activity can result, ultimately, in decreased production of angiotensin II. The use of thiazide diuretics, ACE inhibitors, and ARBs may cause increases in plasma renin activity (see *Chapter 5*). Consequently, inhibition of renin activity may be a potentially effective therapeutic strategy for inhibition of the RAAS. Aliskiren (Tekturna), the first in the new class of direct renin inhibitors, was approved for the treatment of hypertension (**Table 7.14**). It has better oral bioavailability than earlier renin inhibitors and a long plasma half-life that makes it suitable for once-daily dosing.

The use of aliskiren effectively lowers BP both as monotherapy and in combination with a thiazide diuretic (hydrochlorothiazide), an ACE inhibitor (ramipril, lisinopril), an ARB (valsartan), or a CCB (amlodipine). When aliskiren is given with these other antihypertensive agents, plasma renin activity does not increase but remains similar to baseline levels or decreases. Aliskiren has been shown to have a placebolike safety and tolerability profile, and exhibited no interactions with a wide range of commonly used drugs other than furosemide. At the current time, there are limited data on the long-term efficacy and tolerability of aliskiren in the treatment of hypertension in patients with diabetes. Three studies with aliskiren (AVOID, ALOFT, and ALLAY) are ongoing to assess its end-organ protective properties and CHD

TABLE 7.13 — β-Blockers and Combined α_1- and β-Blockers Used in Treating Hypertension[a]

Generic (Trade) Name	Usual Dosage Range (mg)	Frequency	Physiologic Effects	Comments
Atenolol[b] (Tenormin)	25-100	1-2/d	• ↓ Cardiac output	Cardioselective agents may also inhibit β_2-receptors in higher doses (eg, all may aggravate asthma)
Bisoprolol[b] (Zebeta)	2.5-10	1/d	• ↓ Plasma renin activity	
Metoprolol[b] (Lopressor)	50-100	1 or 2/d	• ↓ BP	
Metoprolol XR[b] (Toprol-XL)	50-100	1/d	• ↓ Pulse rate	
Nadolol (Corgard)	40-120	1/d		
Propranolol LA (Inderal LA)	60-180	1/d		
β-Blockers With ISA[c]				
Acebutolol[b] (Sectral)	200-800	2/d	Less effect on heart rate and vascular and bronchial smooth muscle	Possible advantage in subjects with bradycardia who require a β-blocker—they may produce fewer metabolic effects
Penbutolol (Levatol)	10-40	1/d		
Pindolol (Generic)	10-40	2/d		
Combined α_1- and β-Blockers				
Carvedilol (Coreg, Coreg CR)	6.25-25, 10-80	2/d, 1/d	Cardiac output and renal blood flow maintained, BP ↓, *antioxidant effects*	Beneficial effects in HF; may decrease myocardial damage post-MI

Drug	Dose	Frequency	Effects	Comments
Labetalol (Normodyne, Trandate)	200–800	2/d	Cardiac output ± ↓, ↓ plasma renin activity, ↓ BP, some decrease in pulse rate	Probably more effective in blacks than other β-blockers; may cause postural effects; titration should be based on standing BP
Nebivolol (Bystolic)	2.5–40	1/d	Cardiac output maintained, ↓ plasma renin activity, ↓ BP	More effective in blacks than other β-blockers

[a] Dosages may also differ from the manufacturer's prescribing information recommendations. These dosages are based on our experience and the belief that if small or moderate doses of one drug prove ineffective, small doses of a medication from another class should be added.

[b] Cardioselective.

[c] Slight β_2-receptor stimulation.

7

TABLE 7.14 — Renin Inhibitor Used in Treating Hypertension

| Generic (Trade) Name | Usual Dosage | | Adverse Reactions | Physiologic Effects | Comments |
	Range (mg)	Frequency			
Aliskiren (Tekturna)	150-300	1/d	Consistent with AEs of other RAAS inhibitors; generally mild to moderate with incidence similar to placebo	Inhibits production of renin, which cleaves angiotensinogen to AI; reduces plasma renin activity that is increased by treatment with other agents that inhibit the RAAS	As with ACE inhibitors, aliskiren should be discontinued if head or neck angioedema occurs, regardless of severity

outcome. At present, the exact role of this agent has not been determined.

■ Combination Therapy and Combination Agents

In the large clinical trials that have demonstrated that diabetic patients benefit from rigorous lowering of SBP and DBP, at least two or three agents were necessary for optimal BP control. In the UKPDS, approximately two thirds of the type 2 diabetic patients required multiple medications to achieve tight BP control of 144/82 mm Hg. In patients assigned to less-tight control (154/87 mm Hg), there was less-frequent use of multiple antihypertensive agents and less reduction of macrovascular and microvascular risk. The results of this trial indicate that combination therapy with an ACE inhibitor or a β-blocker plus a diuretic is more effective than monotherapy in reducing macrovascular and microvascular events, providing that BP is adequately lowered.

When ACE inhibitors or ARBs are used in conjunction with low-dose diuretics, metabolic problems such as hyperkalemia (which may occur with these agents alone) and hypokalemia/hypomagnesemia (with diuretics) are rare. β-Blockers and low-dose diuretics also may represent good combination therapy in diabetic patients. FACET also provided some support for the use of an ACE inhibitor and CCB as combination therapy. In FACET, the incidence of CVD was less in the group treated with the ACE inhibitor fosinopril than in the group that received the CCB amlodipine, but the incidence of CVD events was least in the group that received both antihypertensive agents (**Figure 7.5**). These results and data from other studies, such as the ACCOMPLISH trial, suggest that ACE inhibitor and CCB combinations are effective in reducing CVD risk in diabetics with evidence of renal disease.

In summary, once baseline ACE inhibitor or ARB therapy has been initiated and if goal BP has not been achieved, then combinations with low-dose diuretics or CCBs represent an appropriate therapeutic approach to accomplish the BP goal of 130/80-85 mm Hg, and thus reduce macrovascular and microvascular disease in this high-risk population. Available combination

FIGURE 7.5 — Major Cardiovascular Events According to Treatment

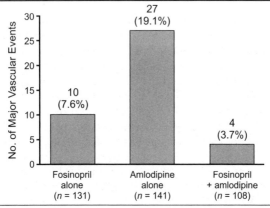

Cardiovascular events were reduced more with an ACE inhibitor than with a CCB in the Fosinopril vs Amlodipine Cardiovascular Event Trial (FACET) in diabetics with evidence of renal disease. Best results were obtained when both agents were given together (small number of events).

Tatti P, et al. *Diabetes Care*. 1998;21:597-603.

hypertensive medications are listed in **Table 7.15**. In many cases, physicians may elect to start therapy in a diabetic hypertensive with a combination of an ACE inhibitor or an ARB plus a diuretic or a CCB. This is the current recommendation of the JNC 7, especially if stage 2 hypertension is present (BP >160/100 mm Hg).

Specific Treatment Plan and Case Presentation

The treatment algorithm (**Figure 7.1**) can be used as a guide to management of the following case of diabetes and hypertension.

■ Case Presentation

A 51-year-old woman with adult-onset (type 2) diabetes of 8 years' duration presented for evaluation and optimization of therapy. Her diabetes was initially controlled on a sulfonylurea drug, but 2 years ago, metformin was added for better blood glucose control. She is overweight at 5'4" and 170 lb (ideal weight would be about 120-130 lb). She has been trying to lose weight, but has gained 2 lb over the past year. Her most recent fasting blood glucose levels are in the range of 110 to 140 mg/dL. Her BP was noted to be elevated 2 years prior to this visit and she has been taking amlodipine 5 mg/day with reported good BP control. She does not remember having her urine checked, having an electrocardiogram (ECG), or having an eye exam. She has a family history of heart disease, kidney disease, and type 2 diabetes. She has gone through menopause over the past year and a half with hot flashes and a discontinuation of menstrual bleeding 6 to 9 months ago. She does not smoke and drinks moderately– one glass of wine every other day.

On physical examination, she is a pleasant, talkative, obese woman with some increase in central distribution of fat. Vital signs include a heart rate of 86 beats per minute and BP of 166/94 mm Hg. Funduscopic exam reveals grade 2 hypertensive changes (A-V nicking) with no evidence of proliferative diabetic retinopathy. There are no carotid bruits and the thyroid is of normal size. Cardiac exam reveals a normal rate and rhythm with an S_4 gallop at the apex, which is 2 cm lateral to the mid-clavicular line. Examination of the abdomen reveals no bruits or other abnormalities. Peripheral pulses are normal and no abnormal neurologic findings are evident.

Initial testing includes an ECG that is normal except for voltage criteria of LVH and a spot urine albumin-to-creatinine level of 3.5 mg/mmol (normal, <2.0). Fasting glucose is 118 mg/dL and a fasting lipid profile reveals total cholesterol of 243 mg/dL, HDL 32 mg/dL, triglycerides 220 mg/dL, and LDL cholesterol 162 mg/dL. Serum creatinine is 1.1 mg/dL, and electrolytes are normal. Goals for this woman's management should include the following:

- In conjunction with a dietitian, a diet should be planned, and increased walking as a suitable form of aerobic exercise encouraged. Since she does not have a history of angina, an exercise ECG test or an exercise thallium scan is not indicated unless she plans to embark on a much more vigorous exercise program.

TABLE 7.15 — Combination Antihypertensive Medications

Generic Name	Trade Name	Available Doses (mg)
ACE Inhibitors and Diuretics		
Benazepril/hydrochlorothiazide	Lotensin HCT	5/6.25, 10/12.5, 20/12.5, 20/25
Captopril/hydrochlorothiazide	Capozide[a]	25/15, 25/25, 50/15, 50/25
Enalapril/hydrochlorothiazide	Vaseretic	5/12.5, 10/25
Fosinopril/hydrochlorothiazide	Monopril HCT	10/12.5, 20/12.5
Lisinopril/hydrochlorothiazide	Prinzide; Zestoretic	10/12.5, 20/12.5, 20/25
Moexipril/hydrochlorothiazide	Uniretic	7.5/12.5, 15/12.5, 15/25
Quinapril/hydrochlorothiazide	Accuretic	10/12.5, 20/12.5, 20/25
ARB and CCB		
Amlodipine/valsartan	Exforge	5/160, 10/160, 5/320, 10/320
Amlodipine/olmesartan medoxomil	Azor	5/20, 10/20, 5/40, 10/40
Telmisartan/amlodipine	Twynsta	40/5, 40/10, 80/5, 80/10
ARB, CCB, and Diuretic		
Amlodipine/valsartan/hydrochlorothiazide	Exforge HCT	5/160/12.5, 10/160/12.5, 5/160/25, 10/160/25, 10/320/25

ARBs and Diuretics

Candesartan cilexetil/hydrochlorothiazide	Atacand HCT	16/12.5, 32/12.5
Eprosartan mesylate/hydrochlorothiazide	Teveten HCT	600/12.5, 600/25
Irbesartan/hydrochlorothiazide	Avalide[a]	150/12.5, 300/12.5, 300/25
Losartan potassium/hydrochlorothiazide	Hyzaar[b]	50/12.5, 100/12.5, 100/25
Olmesartan medoxomil/hydrochlorothiazide	Benicar HCT	20/12.5, 40/12.5, 40/25
Telmisartan/hydrochlorothiazide	Micardis HCT	40/12.5, 80/12.5, 80/25
Valsartan/hydrochlorothiazide	Diovan HCT	80/12.5, 160/12.5, 160/25, 320/12.5, 320/25

β-Adrenergic Blockers and Diuretics

Atenolol/chlorthalidone	Tenoretic	50/25, 100/25
Bisoprolol/hydrochlorothiazide	Ziac[a]	2.5/6.25, 5/6.25, 10/6.25
Metoprolol/hydrochlorothiazide	Lopressor HCT	50/25, 100/25, 100/50
Nadolol/bendroflumethiazide	Corzide	40/5, 80/5
Propranolol (XR)/hydrochlorothiazide	Inderide LA	80/50, 120/50, 160/50
Timolol/hydrochlorothiazide	Timolide	10/25

CCBs and ACE Inhibitors

Amlodipine/benazepril	Lotrel	2.5/10, 5/10, 5/20, 10/20, 5/40, 10/40
Felodipine/enalapril	Lexxel	5/5
Trandolapril/verapamil XR	Tarka	2/180, 1/240, 2/240, 4/240

7

Continued

171

TABLE 7.15 — *Continued*

Generic Name	Trade Name	Available Doses (mg)
Other Combinations		
Amiloride/hydrochlorothiazide	Moduretic	5/50
Amlodipine/atorvastatin	Caduet	2.5/10, 2.5/20, 2.5/40, 5/10, 5/20, 5/40, 5/80, 10/10, 10/20, 10/40, 10/80
Clonidine/chlorthalidone	Clorpres	0.1/15, 0.2/15, 0.3/15
Methyldopa/hydrochlorothiazide	Aldoril	250/15, 250/25, 500/30, 500/50
Prazosin/polythiazide	Minizide	1/0.5, 2/0.5, 5/0.5
Reserpine/chlorthalidone	Diupres	250/0.125, 500/0.125
Reserpine/thiazide	Hydropres	25/0.125, 50/0.125
Spironolactone/hydrochlorothiazide	Aldactazide	25/25, 50/50
Triamterene/hydrochlorothiazide	Dyazide	37.5/25
	Maxzide	37.5/25, 75/50

a Approved for initial therapy.
b Approved for initial therapy of severe hypertension (DBP ≥110 mm Hg).

- If she can tolerate aspirin, she should be placed on a minimal dose of 81 mg of aspirin daily.
- Since diet and exercise will lower her LDL by only about 25% at a maximum, or to levels of about 120-130 mg/dL, she should be placed on a 3-hydroxy-3-methylglutaryl coenzyme A (HMG-CoA) reductase inhibitor with the goal of lowering her LDL to <100 mg/dL.
- Given her inadequate BP control, LVH, and albuminuria, she should be placed on an ACE inhibitor or an ARB, which should be titrated at least once if no side effects occur. As she has previously been taking amlodipine, it would be appropriate to continue that along with the ACE inhibitor. Given her relatively high SBP, a third agent (low-dose diuretic) will probably be needed to lower the SBP to ≤130 mm Hg and to reduce albuminuria. It would be appropriate to check the creatinine and potassium 2 to 4 weeks after initiating ACE inhibitor therapy. A slight rise in creatinine at 2 to 4 weeks might occur, but unless there is severe volume depletion or in the rare case where the patient has renal artery stenosis, the creatinine level should not rise significantly and should return to baseline or below the initial level over time. The increase in ACE inhibitor or ARB dosages and the addition of other agents may be accomplished over 1 to 2 months. It would be useful for the physician and educational for this patient if she would purchase a home BP measurement device and have it and her technique for measuring BP validated by the physician. This usually is motivational to the patient, as is home glucose monitoring, and provides additional data to the physician to assist him/her in adjusting the BP regimen over time.

This multifaceted approach to therapy is of great importance in reducing CV events and renal disease progression. *Glycemic control alone is not enough.*

Bakris GL, Williams M, Dworkin L, et al for the National Kidney Foundation Hypertension and Diabetes Executive Committees Working Group. Preserving renal function in adults with hypertension and diabetes: a consensus approach. *Am J Kidney Dis*. 2000;36:646-661.

Bakris GL, Fonseca V, Katholi RE, et al; GEMINI Investigators. Metabolic effects of carvedilol vs metoprolol in patients with type 2 diabetes mellitus and hypertension: a randomized controlled trial. *JAMA*. 2004;292:2227-2236.

Ernst M, Moser M. Use of diuretics in patients with hypertension. *N Engl J Med*. 2009;361:2153-2164.

Gress TW, Nieto FJ, Shahar E, Wofford MR, Brancati FL. Hypertension and antihypertensive therapy as risk factors for type 2 diabetes mellitus. Atherosclerosis Risk in Communities Study. *N Engl J Med*. 2000;342:905-912.

Grundy SM, Benjamin IJ, Burke GL, et al. Diabetes and cardiovascular disease: a statement for healthcare professionals from the American Heart Association. *Circulation*. 1999;100:1134-1146.

Jamerson K, Weber MA, Bakris GL, et al; for the ACCOMPLISH Trial Investigators. Benazepril plus amlodipine or hydrochlorothiazide for hypertension in high-risk patients. *N Engl J Med*. 2008;359:2417-2428.

Lindholm LH, Ibsen H, Dahlof B, et al for the LIFE Study Group. Cardiovascular morbidity and mortality in patients with diabetes in the Losartan Intervention for Endpoint Reduction in Hypertension study (LIFE): a randomised trial against atenolol. *Lancet*. 2002;359:1004-1010.

Moser M. Diuretics and new onset diabetes: is it a problem? *J Hypertens*. 2005;23:666-668.

Moser M. Drug treatment of hypertension in the elderly and in diabetics. In: Van Zwieten PA, Greenlee WJ, eds. *Antihypertensive Drugs*. The Netherlands: Haswood Academic Publishers; 1997.

Moser M. Treating hypertension: calcium channel blockers, diuretics, beta-blockers, ACE inhibitors. Is there a difference? *J Clin Hypertens*. 2000;2:301-304.

Moser M. Is new-onset diabetes of clinical significance in treated hypertensive patients?–Con. *J Clin Hypertens (Greenwich)*. 2006;8:126-132.

Moser M, Falkner B, Weber MA, Keilson LM. The metabolic syndrome–what is it and how should it be managed? *J Clin Hypertens (Greenwich)*. 2006;8:44-49.

Moser M, Sowers J, Giles T. Roundtable discussion: management of hypetension in diabetics. *J Clin Hypertens (Greenwich)*. 2003;5:345-349.

Pool JL, Schmieder RE, Azizi M, et al. Aliskiren, an orally effective renin inhibitor, provides antihypertensive efficacy alone and in combination with valsartan. *Am J Hypertens*. 2007;20:11-20.

O'Brien E, Barton J, Nussberger J, et al. Aliskiren reduces blood pressure and suppresses plasma renin activity in combination with a thiazide diuretic, an angiotensin-converting enzyme inhibitor, or an angiotensin receptor blocker. *Hypertension*. 2007;49:276-284.

Sowers JR. Treatment of hypertension in patients with diabetes. *Arch Intern Med*. 2004;164:1850-1857.

Sowers JR, Reed J. 1999 clinical advisory treatment of hypertension and diabetes. *J Clin Hypertens*. 2000;2:132-133.

The Seventh Report of the Joint National Committee on prevention, detection, evaluation, and treatment of high blood pressure. *JAMA*. 2003;289:2560-2572.

Wright JT, Probsfield JL, Cushman WC, et al; for the ALLHAT Collaborative Research Group. ALLHAT findings revisited in the context of subsequent analyses, other trials, and meta-analyses. *Arch Intern Med*. 2009;169:832-842.

Vaidyanathan S, Valencia J, Kemp C, et al. Lack of pharmacokinetic interactions of aliskiren, a novel direct rennin inhibitor for the treatment of hypertension, with the antihypertensives amlodipine, valsartan, hydrochlorothiazide (HCTZ) and ramipril in healthy volunteers. *Int J Clin Pract*. 2006;60:1343-1356.

7

8

Lipid-Lowering Therapy and Diabetes: Cardiovascular Risk Reduction

Diabetic subjects without a prior myocardial infarction (MI) have almost the same risk of death as nondiabetic individuals who previously have had an MI; an aggressive approach to the management of all known risk factors is therefore warranted. Dyslipidemia should be one of the targets of therapy. The nature of the metabolic defects in lipid and lipoprotein metabolism differs between types 1 and 2 diabetes. The most typical lipoprotein pattern observed in type 2 diabetes consists of:

- Decreased HDL levels (<45 mg/dL)
- High-normal or slightly elevated LDL levels
- Hypertriglyceridemia, usually due to elevated triglyceride-rich, VLDL levels
- Increased small, dense LDL particles and increased intermediate-density lipoprotein (IDL) particles, both of which contribute disproportionately to atherogenic risk
- Total cholesterol, usually normal to slightly elevated.

A similar lipoprotein pattern can be seen in type 1 diabetic patients with nephropathy and in some patients after weight gain in association with intensive insulin treatment. Treated type 1 diabetic patients often have normal lipids and lipoproteins, although hypertriglyceridemia may be the result of inadequate glycemic control.

A major cause of hypertriglyceridemia in treated type 2 diabetic patients is an overproduction of VLDL. Low HDL cholesterol levels are partly due to a replacement of cholesterol in the core of HDL by triglycerides when hypertriglyceridemia is present. HDL levels also may be decreased as a result of impaired catabolism of VLDL. Both LDL and HDL particles are altered by hepatic lipase that is essential for triglyceride catabolism and for normal

HDL production. Reduced activity of lipoprotein lipase is an important cause of hypertriglyceridemia in untreated patients. Complications such as nephropathy and the nephrotic syndrome can alter plasma lipid and lipoprotein levels, with resultant elevations of total cholesterol.

Because of the atherogenic lipid profile of diabetic patients and their higher risk for CVD, all type 2 diabetic patients should be screened for lipid abnormalities at the initial evaluation using a fasting lipid profile to determine serum total cholesterol, triglycerides, and HDL cholesterol. LDL cholesterol is then calculated from the formula: LDL = total cholesterol minus HDL minus (triglycerides divided by 5) if triglycerides are <400 mg/dL (otherwise the formula is inaccurate). All adult type 2 diabetic patients should have their LDL cholesterol lowered to <100 mg/dL, their HDL raised to >45 mg/dL, and triglycerides lowered to <150 mg/dL, if at all possible. This goal is similar to the secondary prevention goal in patients with known CVD. However, an addendum to the National Cholesterol Education Program (NCEP)/Adult Treatment Panel III (ATP III) Guidelines recommends reducing LDL goals to <70 mg/dL for very high-risk and <100 for moderately high-risk patients. Thus in diabetic patients with CV disease, or other high risk factors such as hypertension, a more suitable LDL cholesterol goal should be as close to <70 mg/dL as possible.

Abnormal lipid levels have been identified as having a major impact on events related to atherosclerosis; levels that may be of limited significance in a nondiabetic may be of great significance in a diabetic. IRAS, which included patients with type 2 diabetes with both impaired and normal glucose tolerance, confirmed that dyslipidemia is a greater risk factor for atherosclerosis in diabetics than nondiabetics. Although associations were found between lipoprotein concentrations and internal and common carotid artery thickness, these associations did not substantially differ among persons with and without diabetes. However, while the event rate in nondiabetics is about 10 to 15 CV events per 10,000 person-years with a cholesterol level of about 210 mg/dL, a total cholesterol level of the same magnitude would translate into about 75 events per 10,000 person-years in a diabetic.

Approach to Prevention and Management of Atherosclerosis in Diabetes

The treatment of dyslipidemia in diabetes consists in part of improvement in diabetic control with diet, exercise, and pharmacologic therapy. The NCEP has published dietary recommendations that involve the restriction of dietary fat and cholesterol (**Table 8.1**). This diet, which also utilizes salt restriction, could be considered to be a relatively heart-smart diet for diabetics.

TABLE 8.1 — Diet Recommendations for the Treatment of Lipid Disorders in Diabetes

- Calorie restriction for weight loss as indicated
- Total fat intake <30% of kcal, mostly monounsaturated (eg, canola oil, olive oil)[a]
- Saturated fat intake <7% of total kcal
- Total cholesterol intake <200 mg/d
- Carbohydrate intake 50% to 60% of total calories, emphasizing complex carbohydrates (at least five portions per day of fruits/vegetables); soluble fibers (legumes, oats, certain fruits/vegetables) have additional benefits on total cholesterol, LDL cholesterol level, and glycemic control
- Sodium restriction <2400 mg/d for type 2 diabetic patients with hypertension; sodium restriction <2000 mg/d for type 2 diabetic patients with hypertension and nephropathy

[a] A reduction of total fat to <20% to 25% of total calories is achievable and probably a better target than 30% of total calories on a 2000-calorie/d diet. This suggests an intake of 400 to 500 calories as fat or between 45 and 55 g/fat/d (eg, 45×9 calories/g of fat=405 calories). Food labels will help to guide this level of intake.

In view of the important role of lipids and lipoproteins in CVD and their frequent derangement in diabetes, it is not surprising that aggressive lipid management of the diabetic patient has been associated with a reduction in clinical events in patients with preexisting CVD. A major benefit appears to result from the use of HMG-CoA reductase inhibitors (statins), despite the fact that LDL levels, the lipid fraction primarily affected by these agents, are not usually increased in diabetics. Subgroup analysis of clinical trials in which statins have been used indicate that the reduction in events with statins is at least as great in diabetic as in nondiabetic subjects. Reducing lipid levels (if elevated) has been shown to improve CVD outcomes in diabetic patients. Treatment strategies for lipid abnormalities are reviewed here.

Clinical Trials of Lipid Lowering in Diabetic Subjects

Although few clinical trials have been performed in diabetic subjects specifically to assess the effects of lipid-lowering agents on subsequent coronary heart disease (CHD) events, a number of clinical trials have included a number of patients with type 2 diabetes. **Table 8.2** summarizes the results of various intervention studies to lower lipids in patients with diabetes. These and other trials are discussed below.

■ Statin Trials

In the Scandinavian Simvastatin Survival Study (4S), simvastatin (Zocor) (HMG-CoA reductase inhibitor or statin) significantly reduced CHD incidence and total mortality (borderline significance) in diabetic subjects with high LDL cholesterol and with previous clinical CHD (**Figure 8.1**). Although only 202 patients with diabetes were included in the 4S, simvastatin reduced major coronary events by 55% in the diabetic group and brought about reductions in total cholesterol of 27%; in LDL cholesterol, by 36%; and triglycerides by 11%; HDL cholesterol was increased by 7%.

The Cholesterol and Recurrent Events (CARE) study, which included 586 patients with diabetes, demonstrated that pravastatin (Pravachol) substantially reduced the incidence of a coronary event by 25% in patients with diabetes compared with 23% in those without diabetes. In this study, pravastatin reduced CHD incidence significantly in diabetic subjects with average LDL levels and with previous clinical CHD.

Thus, both 4S and CARE showed substantial benefits of statin therapy in the diabetic population with evidence of CHD. The results indicate that the effect of LDL cholesterol lowering on the risk of death, major CHD events, and any atherosclerotic event is similar in diabetic and nondiabetic patients with CHD. Because the risk of recurrent events is greater in diabetic than in nondiabetic patients with CHD, the absolute clinical benefit achieved by LDL cholesterol lowering may be greater in diabetic patients with CHD.

The Long-Term Intervention With Pravastatin in Ischaemic Disease (LIPID) trial included 782 diabetics. Among the diabetic subgroup, nonfatal MI and death due to CHD were significantly reduced by 19% compared with 25% for nondiabetics. Pravastatin treatment also reduced hospitalization for unstable angina in diabetic patients but to a somewhat lesser degree than in nondiabetic subjects. In the Air Force/Texas Coronary Atherosclerosis Prevention Study (AFCAPS/TexCAPS) primary prevention trial with lovastatin, the reduction of CVD events was significantly greater in the diabetic cohort.

The Heart Protection Study (HPS) enrolled 20,546 high-risk patients of whom 5963 had diabetes with or without CHD or other occlusive arterial disease. Patients were randomized to 5 years of treatment with simvastatin 40 mg daily or placebo. In the total study population, simvastatin treatment decreased coronary mortality by 20% and first nonfatal MI by 37%. There was a 24% reduction in nonfatal and fatal strokes. Allocation to the statin produced a 19% reduction in peripheral macrovascular complications, defined as any peripheral artery surgery, angioplasty, leg amputation, or leg ulcer. In a subgroup, 1981 diabetics had experienced a prior MI or other CHD event. In these patients there was a significant decrease in the occurrence of a new major vascular event in those patients who received a statin (**Figure 8.2**) In the 3982 diabetics with no prior CHD history as well as in the total diabetics (with and without prior MI), there also was a significant reduction in CV events (**Figure 8.2**). These positive results of cholesterol-lowering therapies were achieved with statins in addition to other treatments (ie, ACE inhibitors, β-blockers, and aspirin). The benefits extended to subjects with relatively normal LDL levels

TABLE 8.2 — Four Large-Scale Studies With High Prevalence of Diabetes

Study (N)	Intervention	Primary End Point	Studies Designed to Have Statistical Power	End Point Results Primary	End Point Results Secondary
CARDS (2838 without CHD; 40-75 yo; all type 2 diabetes)	Atorvastatin 10 mg vs placebo	First occurrence of acute CHD events, coronary revascularization, or stroke	90% power to detect a reduction of one third in the primary end point in the atorvastatin 10 mg/d group at a significant level of $P < 0.05$	ARR 0.92% (significant at $P=0.001$); RRR 37%; study stopped at 3.9 years by data and safety monitoring committee due to positive results	Acute CHD events reduced by 36% (−55 to −9); coronary revascularizations by 31% (−59 to 16), and rate of stroke by 48% (−69 to −11). Atorvastatin reduced the death rate by 27% (−48 to 1, $P=0.059$)
FIELD (7664 without CHD, 2131 with previous CVD; 50-75 yo; all type 2 diabetes)	Fenofibrate 200 mg daily vs placebo	In December 2002, the primary end point for the study was amended from CHD death to CHD events (CHD death plus nonfatal MI)	80% power to detect a 22% reduction in CHD events based on an ITT method of analysis	ARR 0.7%; RRR 11%; NS	Significant 24% reduction in nonfatal MI ($P=0.01$) and a NS increase in CHD mortality (1.19, 0.90-1.57; $P=0.22$). Total CVD events significantly reduced from 13.9% to 12.5% (0.89,

Study	Intervention	Outcome	Power	Results	Findings
					0.80-0.99; P=0.035). Also a 21% significant reduction in coronary revascularization (0.79, 0.68-0.93; P= 0.003). Total mortality was 6.6% in the placebo group and 7.3% in the fenofibrate group (P=0.18)
HPS (main study with 20,536 subjects of which 5963 had diabetes: UK adults 40-80 yo)	Simvastatin 40 mg vs placebo	For subgroup analyses for fatal or nonfatal vascular events	>90% power to achieve (P<0.01) a reduced 5-year CHD mortality of about 25% and all-cause mortality by about 15%	ARR 4.9%; RRR 22%; highly significant at P<0.001	18% proportional reduction in CHD death rate; 25% reductions in nonfatal or fatal MI, fatal or nonfatal stroke, and coronary or noncoronary revascularization. Among diabetics, rate of first vascular event reduced by 25%
VA-HIT (2531 men with CHD [VA study]; 550 diabetics by history)	Gemfibrozil 600 mg bid vs placebo	Nonfatal MI or death from coronary causes	90% power to detect a 20% reduction in the primary outcomes with a P<0.05	ARR 4.4%; RRR 22%; highly significant at P=0.006	24% reduction in the combined outcome of death from CHD, nonfatal MI, and stroke (P<0.001). NS differences in the rates of coro-

Continued

8

TABLE 8.2 — *Continued*

Study (N)	Intervention	Primary End Point	Studies Designed to Have Statistical Power	End Point Results Primary	End Point Results Secondary
					nary revascularization, hospitalization for unstable angina, death from any cause, and cancer

Colhoun HM, et al. *Lancet.* 2004;364:685-696; Keech A, et al. *Lancet.* 2005;366:1849-1861; Collins R, et al. *Lancet.* 2003;361:2005-2016; Rubins HB, et al. *N Engl J Med.* 1999;341:410-418.

FIGURE 8.1 — Simvastatin vs Placebo: Curves for Probability of Remaining Free of a Major Coronary Heart Disease Event

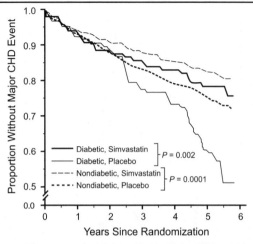

Survival curves for the probability of remaining free of a major CHD event during follow-up in nondiabetic and diabetic patients treated with placebo or simvastatin. The Scandinavian Simvastatin Survival Study (4S) of patients with CHD. Note greater chance of survival without CHD event in both diabetics and nondiabetics in treated groups.

Pyörälä K, et al. *Diabetes Care*. 1997;20:614-620.

<116 mg/dL to both men and women and diabetic patients >65 years of age at entry.

ASCOT was designed to assess whether any synergistic effects were apparent between lipid-lowering and blood-pressure–lowering regimens in preventing CV events. The trial was composed of two arms, the blood-pressure–lowering arm (ASCOT-BPLA) and the lipid-lowering arm (ASCOT-LLA). The results of ASCOT-BPLA are discussed in *Chapter 6*. In the ASCOT-LLA, there were 10,305 subjects, of whom 2532 were diabetics, with a total cholesterol of <252 mg/dL and three additional CVD risk factors. Patients were randomized to receive atorvastatin 10 mg daily or placebo. ASCOT-LLA was stopped prematurely (at a median of 3.3 years of follow-up) due to a significant

FIGURE 8.2 — Effects of Simvastatin Therapy Compared With Placebo on First Major Vascular Event in Different Prior Disease Categories

Prior Disease Category	Simvastatin-Allocated Total Patients/ Incidence (%)	Placebo-Allocated Number/ Incidence (%)
Prior MI or Other CHD + diabetes mellitus	325/972 (33.4)	381/1009 (37.8)
No Prior CHD + diabetes mellitus	276/2006 (13.8)	367/1976 (18.6)
CHD or No Prior CHD + diabetes mellitus	601/2978 (20.2)	748/2985 (25.1)

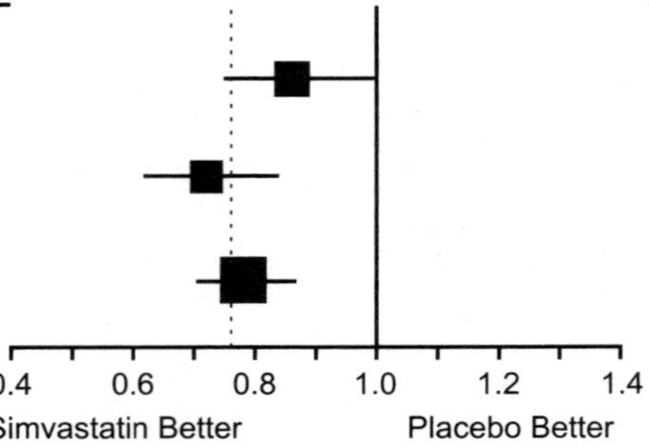

Simvastatin Better   Placebo Better

Adapted from: Heart Protection Study Collaborative Group. *Lancet.* 2002;360:7-22.

37% relative risk reduction in the primary end point in subjects receiving atorvastatin compared with placebo (1.9% vs 3.0%, P <0.001). There was no difference in overall mortality or CV mortality, although it must be noted that the premature termination for efficacy may have prevented attainment of this end point that might have been reached if the trial had been allowed to run for the allotted time. Importantly, in the shorter trial time, ASCOT-LLA demonstrated a significant 27% reduction in fatal and nonfatal stroke (1.7% vs 2.4%, P = 0.02).

In the Collaborative Atorvastatin Diabetes Study (CARDS), 2838 patients with type 2 diabetes, low LDL cholesterol concentration ($\leq$159.8 mg/dL), low fasting triglyceride level ($\leq$600 mg/dL), but with at least one other risk factor for but no prior CVD, were randomized to atorvastatin 10 mg daily or placebo. The study was stopped 2 years earlier than expected (mean follow-up 3.9 years) because the prespecified early stopping rule for efficacy had been met. Patients treated with atorvastatin had a 36% reduction in acute coronary events and a 48% reduction in stroke compared with patients who were not treated with atorvastatin (**Figure 8.3**). These observations indicate that most patients with diabetes should be given a statin, even if their LDL cholesterol is not at levels considered to be elevated.

The potential benefit of treating patients even with low levels of LDL cholesterol is also supported by the results of the Study to Evaluate the Effect of Rosuvastatin on Intravascular Ultrasound-Derived Coronary Atheroma Burden (ASTEROID) study, which used intravascular ultrasound (IVUS) to assess the effect of very intensive statin therapy with rosuvastatin 40 mg daily on changes in coronary atheroma burden. A total of 349 patients with CHD had evaluable serial IVUS examinations at baseline and after 24 months of treatment. The mean LDL level declined from 130.4 mg/dL at baseline to 60.8 mg/dL, a reduction of 53.2% (P <0.001). Mean HDL increased from 43.1 mg/dL at baseline to 49.0 mg/dL, an increase of 14.7% (P <0.001). The percent atheroma volume for the entire vessel decreased by 3.15%, (P <0.001 vs baseline) and the total atheroma volume was reduced by 6.8% (P <0.001 vs baseline). These results also appear

8

FIGURE 8.3 — Cumulative Hazard of Primary End Point, All-Cause Mortality, and Any Cardiovascular End Point[a]: CARDS

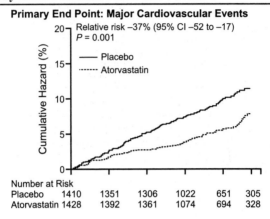

Primary End Point: Major Cardiovascular Events

Relative risk –37% (95% CI –52 to –17)
P = 0.001

—— Placebo
------ Atorvastatin

Number at Risk						
Placebo	1410	1351	1306	1022	651	305
Atorvastatin	1428	1392	1361	1074	694	328

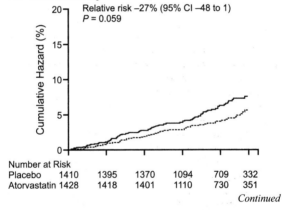

All-Cause Mortality

Relative risk –27% (95% CI –48 to 1)
P = 0.059

Number at Risk						
Placebo	1410	1395	1370	1094	709	332
Atorvastatin	1428	1418	1401	1110	730	351

Continued

to indicate that intensive treatment of patients with evidence of CHD and LDL levels that are not considered to be elevated, when accompanied by significant HDL increases, can result in regression of atherosclerosis in patients with CHD. Since diabetics without CHD often have the same CV event risk as nondiabetics with CHD, these results are probably applicable to diabetic individuals, especially if they are hypertensive.

A recent meta-analysis compared results of statin therapy in 18,000 diabetic patients with results in a non-

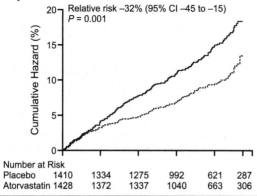

Any Cardiovascular End Point

Type of First Event	Placebo ($n=1410$)	Atorvastatin ($n=1428$)
Fatal MI	20	8
Other acute CHD death	4	10
Nonfatal MI[a]	41	25
Unstable angina	9	7
Resuscitated cardiac arrest	0	0
Coronary revascularization	18	12
Fatal stroke	5	1
Nonfatal stroke	30	20
TOTAL	127	83

P for heterogeneity.

[a] Five silent MIs included in each group.

Colhoun HM, et al. *Lancet.* 2004;364:685-696.

diabetic group. Results were similar, with a significant reduction in all-cause and vascular mortality.

■ **Fibrate Trials**

A number of studies have been performed using fibrates, such as gemfibrozil (Lopid) or fenofibrate (Tricor), which theoretically may be more ideally suited to use in diabetic dyslipidemia. These studies have indicated that fibrates have a beneficial effect in diabetic subjects.

In the Helsinki Heart Study, gemfibrozil (fibric acid derivative) was associated with a nonstatistically significant reduction in CHD in diabetic subjects without prior

CHD. In the Veterans Affairs High-Density Lipoprotein Cholesterol Intervention Trial (VA-HIT), gemfibrozil was associated with a 24% decrease in CV events in diabetic subjects with CVD.

The Diabetes Atherosclerosis Intervention Study (DAIS) was the first trial in people with type 2 diabetes specifically designed to ascertain the effects of correcting lipoprotein abnormalities on the progression or regression of coronary atherosclerosis. The 418 study subjects were followed for >3 years at 11 centers in Canada, Finland, France, and Sweden. All patients had lipid profiles typical of their condition: mild elevations of plasma triglycerides (mean, 214 mg/dL) and LDL (mean, 133 mg/dL), and a high ratio of total cholesterol to HDL (215 mg/dL/39 mg/dL = 5.5). Nearly half of the patients had a history of CHD, and a third had undergone a prior coronary intervention. At baseline, all subjects underwent coronary angiography to ensure that they had at least one measurable lesion. They were then randomized to fenofibrate (200 mg/day) or placebo and followed for 3 years.

Upon completion of treatment, all patients underwent coronary angiography to measure the progression of atherosclerosis. Fenofibrate treatment was shown to reduce triglycerides, total cholesterol, and LDL, and to increase levels of HDL; notably, these results occurred in a population whose lipid levels were on average only slightly abnormal (**Figure 8**.**4**). In a subgroup of patients (one third of the total population)—with the most abnormal levels—triglycerides were reduced by 39%, LDL was reduced by 15%, and HDL was increased by 6.3%. In comparison with the placebo-treated group, patients treated with fenofibrate had a 40% reduction in the rate of progression of localized lesions. These changes were directly related to the lipid levels attained during the treatment period. CHD progression was reduced in both men and women, as well as in patients with and without a history of prior coronary interventions. There was also an accompanying 23% reduction in combined CHD events. Thus this study provided good evidence that correcting (or even partially correcting) the lipid abnormalities in diabetic subjects is beneficial and that medication other than a statin can be effective.

FIGURE 8.4 — Changes in Lipid Values From Baseline in Placebo and Fenofibrate Groups

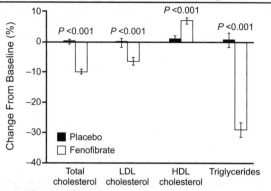

Diabetes Atherosclerosis Intervention Study Investigators. *Lancet.* 2001;357:907.

The Fenofibrate Intervention and Event Lowering in Diabetes (FIELD) study was a randomized, controlled trial in patients with type 2 diabetes who were not taking statin therapy at study entry. After a placebo and a fenofibrate run-in phase, 9795 patients (2131 with previous CV disease and 7664 without) with a total-cholesterol concentration of 115-250 mg/dL and a total-cholesterol/HDL-cholesterol ratio of ≥4.0 or plasma triglyceride of 88.5-442.5 mg/dL were randomized to fenofibrate 200 mg/day ($n=4895$) or matching placebo ($n=4900$). The diabetics randomized to fenofibrate therapy had a statistically insignificant mean risk reduction of 11% in the primary outcome, ie, incidence overall of CHD death or nonfatal MI. However, this same group demonstrated statistically significant changes in the secondary end point of total CVD events with a significant 11% risk reduction ($P=0.035$). Many subjects in the placebo group were given statins by their physicians. The study authors speculated that the higher rate of starting statin therapy in patients allocated to placebo might have masked a moderately larger treatment benefit.

Further analyses of results in type 2 diabetics in the FIELD trial reported that the use of a fenofibrate resulted in a significant reduction of clinical and silent

MIs by 19% ($P=0.006$) and nonfatal clinical MIs by 24% ($P=0.01$), with a nonstatistically significant reduction of 16% ($P=0.16$) in silent MIs. Overall, >36% of the MIs were silent, a finding not unusual in type 2 diabetics. Subsequent MIs in the silent MI group were, however, significantly reduced.

Another observation in the FIELD trial was the finding that fenofibrate increased serum creatinine levels. This increase was abrogated when fenofibrate was discontinued, suggesting that the impact was on reno-hemodynamics. Practitioners need to be aware of this effect, particularly when diabetic hypertensive patients are receiving RAAS blockers or metformin.

Treatment of Dyslipidemia in Diabetic Patients

Weight reduction and increased physical activity may lead to decreased triglycerides and increased HDL levels and also to a modest lowering of LDL cholesterol levels. Diabetic patients who are overweight should be given instructions on diet and increased physical activity. As noted, the proportion of saturated fat should be reduced. The ADA suggests an increase either in carbohydrate or in monounsaturated fat to compensate for the reduction in saturated fat (ie, cut down on fatty meats, butter, eggs, etc). Some (but not all) studies suggest that a high monounsaturated or polyunsaturated fat diet (more fish, olive oil, etc) may have better metabolic effects than a high-carbohydrate diet, although other experts have suggested that such a dietary modification may make weight loss more difficult in obese diabetic patients.

Recommendations of the American Heart Association (AHA) for patients with CHD indicate that adherence to a diet typically reduces LDL cholesterol by about 15-25 mg/dL. Thus if the LDL level exceeds the goal by >25 mg/dL or if the patient is unlikely to follow the prescribed diet, the physician should probably institute pharmacologic therapy at the same time as behavioral therapy in high-risk patients (ie, diabetic patients) to achieve LDL levels <100 mg/dL. In other patients, dietary interventions may be evaluated at 6-week intervals with consideration of pharmacologic therapy after 3 and 6 months.

Generally, pharmacologic therapy is instituted along with diet therapy for the aggressive correction of abnormal lipid levels in patients with diabetes. A mainstay of therapy is a statin (eg, atorvastatin, fluvastatin, lovastatin, pravastatin, rosuvastatin, or simvastatin). These drugs inhibit cholesterol synthesis, up-regulate LDL receptors, and may help stabilize vulnerable atherosclerotic plaques, which are more prevalent and lethal in patients with diabetes. If additional triglyceride lowering is indicated, a fibric acid derivative such as fenofibrate can be added.

As both statins and fibrates have been shown to reduce the risk of CV events, the use of combination therapy may achieve additional risk reduction over and above that achieved with statin monotherapy. Because the combination is more likely to cause liver function abnormalities as well as myopathies, creatine phosphokinase (CPK) and liver function should be monitored more closely. Once a stable and effective dose of the combination is reached and CPK and liver function tests are less than three times the upper limit of normal, monitoring becomes less necessary. Dosing information on these lipid-lowering drugs is presented in **Table 8.3**.

While niacin is the most effective drug for raising HDL, in high doses it may raise blood glucose and cause disturbing side effects (eg, headaches and flushing). Smaller doses (750-2000 mg/day), however, have been shown to have beneficial effects on LDL, HDL, and triglycerides with only small changes in blood glucose. These are generally responsive to adjustment of diabetic therapy. Combination therapy, with a statin and a fibrate, statin, or niacin, may be efficacious for patients needing treatment for all three lipid functions.

While the primary goal of statin and fibrate therapy in diabetic patients is to correct dyslipidemia, the results of an 8-year observational study in Australia showed that treatment of diabetic patients with either a statin or fibrate reduced the risk of developing peripheral neuropathy by 35% and 48%, respectively. Although these results are encouraging, this was an observational study and not

TABLE 8.3 — Lipid-Lowering Drugs: Preparations and Usual Dosing Regimens

Drug (Trade Name)	Availability	Starting Dose	Dose Range
Cholestyramine (Questran, Questran Light, Prevalite)	Powder for Oral Suspension: single-dose (4 g) packets or cans with dosing scoop (1 scoop=1 dose)	4 g/d (1 scoop)	4-12 g bid
Colestipol (Colestid)	Granules: single-dose (5 g) packets or bottles with dosing scoop (1 scoop=1 dose)	5 g/d (1 scoop)	5-15 g bid
	Tablet: 1 g		
Colesevelam (WelChol)	Tablet: 625 mg	6 tablets/d	7 tablets/d (qd or bid)
Ezetimibe (Zetia)	Tablet: 10 mg	10 mg/d	10 mg/d
Gemfibrozil (Lopid)	Tablet: 600 mg	600 mg bid	600 mg bid
Fenofibrates:			
(Antara)	Capsule: 43, 87, 130 mg	43-130 mg/d	43-130 mg/d
(Lofibra)	Capsule: 67, 134, 200 mg	67-200 mg/d	67-200 mg/d
(TriCor)	Tablet: 48, 145 mg	48-145 mg/d	48-145 mg/d
(Triglide)	Tablet: 50, 160 mg	50-160 mg/d	60-160 mg/d
(Trilipix)	Capsule: 45, 135 mg	45-135 mg/d	45-135 mg/d
Nicotinic acid:			
Immediate-release (Niacor, others)	Tablet: 5, 100, 250, 500, 1000 mg	50 mg tid	500-2000 mg tid
Sustained-release (Niaspan, others)	Tablet: 250, 375, 500, 750, 1000 mg	500 mg/d	1000-2000 mg/d

n-3 Fatty acids:			
Unfractionated fish oils	Capsule: 1 g	3 g tid	2-6 g tid
n-3 Fatty acid ethyl esters (Lovaza)	Capsule: 1 g	1-2 g bid	2-3 g bid
HMG-CoA Reductase Inhibitors			
Atorvastatin (Lipitor)	Tablet: 10, 20, 40, 80 mg	10 mg/d	10-80 mg/d
Fluvastatin (Lescol)	Capsule: 20, 40 mg	20-40 mg qpm	20-40 mg qpm,
(Lescol XL)	Tablet, ER: 80		40 mg bid; for ER tablet, 80 mg qpm
Lovastatin (Altocor)	Tablet, ER: 10, 20, 40, 60 mg	20 mg qpm	10-40 mg qpm,
(Mevacor)	Tablet: 10, 20, 40 mg	20 mg qpm	40 mg bid
Pravastatin (Pravachol)	Tablet: 10, 20, 40, 80 mg	40 mg qpm	10-80 mg qpm
Rosuvastatin (Crestor)	Tablet: 5, 10, 20, 40 mg	5-20 mg/d	5-40 mg/d
Simvastatin (Zocor)	Tablet: 5, 10, 20, 40, 80 mg	20 mg qpm	5-80 mg qpm
Combinations			
Niacin/Lovastatin (Advicor)	Tablet: 500/20, 750/20, 1000/20, 1000/40 mg	500/20 qhs	500/20-2000/40 mg qhs
Niacin/Simvastatin (Simcor)	Tablet: 500/20, 750/20, 1000/20	500/20 mg/d	500/20-2000/40 mg/d
Ezetimibe/Simvastatin (Vytorin)	Tablet: 10/10, 10/20, 10/40, 10/80 mg	10/20 mg/d	10/10-10/80 mg/d

Key: bid, twice daily; HMG-CoA, 3-hydroxy-3-methylglutaryl coenzyme A; qd, every day; qpm, each evening; qhs, at bedtime; tid, three times a day.

8

an intervention trial. Therefore, the results should be interpreted with some caution.

Treatment Goals for Lipoprotein Therapy

Because of frequent changes in glycemic control in adult diabetic patients and their effects on levels of lipoprotein levels, LDL, HDL, total cholesterol, and triglycerides should be measured every year or more frequently during titration of medications given to correct abnormal levels. If values decrease to goal levels (see below), assessment may be repeated every 18 months to 2 years. In children with diabetes, consideration should be given to measuring lipoproteins after age 2 years, as suggested by the NCEP Reports of the Expert Panel on Blood Cholesterol in Children and Adolescents. Optimal LDL cholesterol levels for adults with diabetes are <70 mg/dL (especially if there is evidence of CHD), optimal HDL cholesterol levels are >45 mg/dL, desirable triglyceride levels are <150 mg/dL, and desirable total cholesterol levels are <200 mg/dL. Nondiabetic women tend to have higher HDL cholesterol levels than men. It may be desirable to have even higher HDL cholesterol levels than 45 mg/dL. However, raising HDL cholesterol levels pharmacologically in diabetic patients is difficult since one of the effective agents for raising HDL levels is nicotinic acid, which, as noted, may actually raise blood glucose levels in diabetic patients. Fibrates may, however, raise HDL levels significantly without affecting glycemic control.

The recommendations for treatment of elevated LDL cholesterol generally follow the guidelines of both the NCEP and an ADA consensus development conference with the following caveats: Pharmacologic therapy should be initiated after behavioral interventions are tried. However, in patients with clinical CVD, pharmacologic therapy with a statin should be initiated at the same time that behavioral therapy is started.

In the context of the NCEP report, it is suggested that after nutrition therapy and glucose interventions, diabetic subjects with clinical CHD and an LDL level >100 mg/

dL should be treated with pharmacologic agents. For diabetic patients without preexisting CHD, the current recommendations for starting pharmacologic therapy are an LDL level of ≥130 mg/dL, with a goal of ≤100 mg/dL (2.60 mmol/L) for LDL (diabetes should be considered a high CHD risk factor) (**Table 8.4**). These recommendations are based not only on the high incidence of CHD in patients with diabetes, but also on their higher fatality rate once they have CHD. Since a large proportion of diabetic patients die from an acute coronary event before they reach the hospital, a preventive strategy based solely on secondary prevention after a CHD event would not be able to "save" large numbers of these diabetic patients. In patients with LDL levels >100 mg/dL, a variety of treatment strategies are available, including more aggressive diet therapy and pharmacologic treatment with a statin. In addition, if the HDL is <40 mg/dL, a fibric acid such as fenofibrate might be used in patients with an LDL between 100 and 129 mg/dL.

New-Onset Diabetes With Statin Therapy—Is It of Significance?

A recent trial (JUPITER) evaluating the use of one of the statins (rosuvastatin) in patients with average LDL levels but elevated levels of high sensitivity CRP reported an absolute increase in the occurrence of NOD of 0.6%, which was statistically significant. Is this finding of clinical significance and consistent with other data? A review of the major studies with statins reveals mixed results with either a minimal or no increase in the development of type 2 diabetes with these medications. The preponderance of evidence suggests that diabetics derive substantial benefit and a decrease in CV events and mortality with corrections of lipid abnormalities. Thus, concern about the slight changes in blood glucose or in the occurrence of NOD with statins should not, at this time, change the approach to lipid-lowering therapy. Efforts to lower LDL and triglycerides while raising HDL levels in diabetic patients or in patients with the metabolic syndrome should be a priority in treatment.

TABLE 8.4 — LDL Cholesterol Goals and End Points for Therapeutic Lifestyle Changes and Drug Therapy in Different Risk Categories[a]

Risk Category	LDL-c Goal	Initiate TLC	Consider Drug Therapy[b]
High Risk			
CHD[a] or CHD risk equivalents[c] (10-year risk >20%)	<100 mg/dL (optional goal: <70 mg/dL)[f]	≥100 mg/dL[d]	≥100mg/dL[e] (<100 mg/dL: consider drug options)[b]
Moderately High Risk			
2+ Risk factors[g] (10-year risk 10%-20%)[i]	<130 mg/dL[h]	≥130 mg/dL[d]	≥130 mg/dL (100-129 mg/dL; consider drug options)[j]
Moderate Risk			
2+ Risk factors[g] (10-year risk <10%)[i]	<130 mg/dL	≥130 mg/dL	≥160 mg/dL
Lower Risk			
0-1 Risk factor[k]	<160 mg/dL	≥160 mg/dL	≥190 mg/dL (160-189 mg/dL: LDL-lowering drug optional)

[a] CHD includes history of MI, unstable angina, stable angina, coronary artery procedures (angioplasty or bypass surgery), or evidence of clinically significant myocardial ischemia.

[b] When LDL-lowering drug therapy is employed, it is advised that intensity of therapy be sufficient to achieve at least a 30% to 40% reduction in LDL-c levels.

c CHD risk equivalents include clinical manifestations of noncoronary forms of atherosclerotic disease (peripheral arterial disease, abdominal aortic aneurysm, and carotid artery disease [transient ischemic attacks or stroke of carotid origin or >50% obstruction of a carotid artery]), diabetes, and 2+ risk factors with 10-year risk for hard CHD >20%.

d Any person at high risk or moderately high risk who has lifestyle-related risk factors (eg, obesity, physical inactivity, elevated tri-glyceride, low HDL-c, or metabolic syndrome) is a candidate for TLC to modify these risk factors regardless of LDL-c level.

e If baseline LDL-c is <100 mg/dL, institution of an LDL-lowering drug is a therapeutic option on the basis of available clinical trial results. If a high-risk person has high triglycerides or low HDL-c, combining a fibrate or nicotinic acid with an LDL-lowering drug can be considered.

f Very high risk favors the optional LDL-c goal of <70 mg/dL, and in patients with high triglycerides, non–HDL-c <100 mg/dL.

g Risk factors include cigarette smoking, hypertension (BP ≥140/90 mm Hg or on antihypertensive medication), low HDL-c (<40 mg/dL), family history of premature CHD (CHD in male first-degree relative <55 yo; CHD in female first-degree relative <65 yo), and age (men ≥45 yo; women ≥55 yo).

h Optional LDL-c goal <100 mg/dL.

i Electronic 10-year risk calculators are available at www.nhlbi.nih.gov/guidelines/cholesterol.

j For moderately high-risk persons, when LDL-c level is 100 to 129 mg/dL, at baseline or on lifestyle therapy, initiation of an LDL-lowering drug to achieve an LDL-c level <100 mg/dL is a therapeutic option on the basis of available clinical trial results.

k Almost all people with no or one risk factor have a 10-year risk <10%, and 10-year risk assessment in people with no or one risk factor is thus not necessary.

Grundy SM, et al. *Circulation.* 2004;110:227-239.

8

Lipid-Lowering Agents

A brief summary of the actions of the available agents for lipid lowering in patients with diabetes is shown in **Table 8.5**, along with the order of priority for treatment. Treatment of high LDL is considered the first priority for pharmacologic therapy of dyslipidemia for a number of reasons. Clinical trials (see previous discussion) have demonstrated the effectiveness of statins in reducing CHD in diabetic subjects. The Helsinki Heart Study, DAIS, and VA-HIT have indicated a reduction in CHD in this patient population with fibrate therapy. The effect of these pharmacologic agents on lipoproteins is summarized in **Table 8.6**. Generally, one or two agents are available in each class of drugs with the exception of the statins. The choice of a statin should depend principally on the LDL reduction needed to achieve the target (<100 mg/dL), the initial LDL level, and the judgment of the treating physician. The effects of the various statins in lower or moderate dosages on LDL, HDL, and triglycerides are summarized in **Table 8.7**.

TABLE 8.5 — Order of Priorities for Treatment of Diabetic Dyslipidemia in Adults

LDL Cholesterol Lowering
- Lifestyle interventions
- Preferred: HMG CoA reductase inhibitor (statin)
- Others: bile acid–binding resin, cholesterol absorption inhibitor, fenofibrate, or niacin

HDL Cholesterol Raising
- Lifestyle interventions
- Nicotinic acid or fibrates

Triglyceride Lowering
- Lifestyle interventions
- Glycemic control
- Fibric acid derivative (fenofibrate, gemfibrozil), niacin, high-dose statins (in those who also have high LDL cholesterol)

Combined Hyperlipidemia
- First choice: improved glycemic control plus high-dose statin
- Second choice: improved glycemic control plus statin plus fibric acid derivative
- Third choice: Improved glycemic control plus statin plus nicotinic acid

Decision for treatment of high LDL cholesterol before elevated triglycerides is based on clinical trial data indicating safety as well as efficacy of the available agents. The combination of statins with nicotinic acid, fenofibrate, or especially gemfibrozil may carry an increased risk of myositis. Patients with triglyceride levels >400 mg/dL require special consideration.

Adapted from: American Diabetes Association. *Diabetes Care.* 2004; 27(suppl 1):S69.

8

TABLE 8.6 — Pharmacologic Agents for Treatment of Dyslipidemia in Adults

	Effect on Lipoprotein			Clinical Trials in
Agent	LDL	HDL	Triglyceride	**Diabetic Subjects**
First-Line Agents for Lowering LDL, Raising HDL, and Decreasing Triglycerides				
LDL-lowering HMG-CoA reductase inhibitor	↓↓	↔↑	↔↓	4S (simvastatin) CARE (pravastatin) CARDS (atorvastatin) HPS (simvastatin)
Fibric acid derivatives	↓↔↑	↑	↓↓	Helsinki (gemfibrozil) DAIS (fenofibrate) VA-HIT (gemfibrozil)
Second-Line Agents				
LDL-lowering bile acid–binding resins	↓	↔	↑	None
LDL- and triglyceride-lowering nicotinic acid[a]	↓	↑↑	↓↓	None

[a] In diabetic patients, nicotinic acid should be restricted to ≤ 2 g/d; short-acting nicotinic acid is preferred.

American Diabetes Association. Physical activity/exercise and type 2 diabetes. *Diabetes Care*. 2006;29:1433-1438.

American Diabetes Association. Standards of medical care in diabetes. *Diabetes Care*. 2009;32(suppl 1):S13-S61.

American Diabetes Association. Nutrition recommendations and interventions for diabetes: a position statement of the American Diabetes Association. *Diabetes Care*. 2007;30:S48-S65.

Athyros VG, Papageorgiou AA, Athyrou VV, Demitriadis DS, Kontopoulos AG. Atorvastatin and micronized fenofibrate alone and in combination in type 2 diabetes with combined hyperlipidemia. *Diabetes Care*. 2002;25:1198-1202.

Bosch J, Lonn E, Pogue J, et al; HOPE/HOPE-TOO Study Investigators. Long-term effects of ramipril on cardiovascular events and on diabetes: results of the HOPE study extension. *Circulation*. 2005;112:1339-1346.

Burgess DC, Hunt D, Li L, et al. Incidence and predictors of silent myocardial infarction in type 2 diabetes and the effect of fenofibrate: an analysis from the Fenofibrate Intervention and Event Lowering in Diabetes (FIELD) study [published online ahead of print September 29, 2009]. *Eur Heart J*. doi:10.1093/eurheartj/ehp377.

Cholesterol Treatment Trialists (CTT) Collaborators; Kearney PM, Blackwell L, Collins R, et al. Efficacy of cholesterol-lowering therapy in 18,686 people with diabetes in 14 randomised trials of statins: a meta-analysis. *Lancet*. 2008;371:117-125.

Colhoun HM, Betteridge DJ, Durrington PN, et al; CARDS investigators. Primary prevention of cardiovascular disease with atorvastatin in type 2 diabetes in the Collaborative Atorvastatin Diabetes Study (CARDS): multicentre randomised placebo-controlled trial. *Lancet*. 2004;364:685-696.

Davis TM, Yeap BB, Davis WA, Bruce DG. Lipid-lowering therapy and peripheral sensory neuropathy in type 2 diabetes: the Fremantle Diabetes Study. *Diabetologia*. 2008;51:562-566.

Diabetes Atherosclerosis Intervention Study Investigators. Effect of fenofibrate on progression of coronary-artery disease in type 2 diabetes: the Diabetes Atherosclerosis Intervention study, a randomised study. *Lancet*. 2001;357:905-910.

Grundy SM, Cleeman JI, Merz CN, et al; National Heart, Lung, and Blood Institute; American College of Cardiology Foundation; American Heart Association. Implications of recent clinical trials for the National Cholesterol Education Program Adult Treatment Panel III guidelines. *Circulation*. 2004;110:227-239.

8

TABLE 8.7 — Efficacy of HMG-CoA Reductase Inhibitors

Drug	Dose (mg/d)	Change (%)		
		LDL-c	HDL-c	TG
Atorvastatin[1]	5	−29	+8	−25
	10	−36	+7	−13
	20	−46	+6	−22
	40	−50	+3	−30
	80	−58	+2	−26
Fluvastatin	20[2]	−21	+3	−8
	40[2]	−26	+3	−12
	80[3a]	−32	—	—
	80[4b]	−34	+8.5	−12.4
Lovastatin[5]	20	−24	+7	−10
	40	−34	+9	−16
	80	−40	+10	−19
Pravastatin	10[6]	−18	+5	−5
	20[7]	−25	+6	−13
	40[8]	−28	+7	−11
	80[9]	−37	+3	−19
Rosuvastatin	5[10]	−42	+8	−16
	10[10]	−47	+9	−19
	20[11]	−52	+10	−20
	40[11]	−57	+10	−23
Simvastatin	5[12]	−23	+8	−10
	10[12]	−28	+6	−9
	20[12]	−37	+6	−12
	40[13]	−40	+12	−19
	80[13]	−46	+4[c]	−19[c]
	80[13]	−46	+10[d]	−36[d]

[a] Administered as 40 mg bid.

[b] Administered as 80-mg sustained-release tablet at bedtime.

[c] TG <200 mg/dL.

[d] TG >200 mg/dL.

1. Data for 5 mg/d (*n* = 13) are taken from Nawrocki JW, et al. *Arterioscler Thromb Vasc Biol*. 1995;15:678-682. Data for 10 mg/d (*n* = 1090) are taken from: (1) Bertolini S et al. *Atherosclerosis*. 1997;130:191-197; (2) Dart A, et al. *Am J Cardiol*. 1997;80:39-44; (3) Davidson M, et al. *Am J Cardiol*. 1997;79:1475-1481; (4) Heinonen TM, et al. *Clin Ther*. 1996;18:853-863; and (5) Nawrocki JW, et al. *Arterioscler Thromb Vasc Biol*. 1995;15:678-682.

Continued

Data for 40 mg/d ($n=26$) are taken from: (1) Cilla DD Jr, et al. *J Clin Pharmacol.* 1996;36:604-609; and (2) Nawrocki JW, et al. *Arterioscler Thromb Vasc Biol.* 1995;15:678-682. Data for 80 mg/d ($n=11$) are taken from Nawrocki JW, et al. *Arterioscler Thromb Vasc Biol.* 1995;15:678-682. Jones P, et al. *Am J Cardiol.* 1998;81:582-587 contributes data for 10, 20, 40, and 80 mg/d.

2. Data for 20 mg/d ($n=1066$) and 40 mg/d ($n=633$) are taken from a summary of blinded, placebo-controlled trials: Peters TK, et al. *Drugs.* 1994;47(suppl 2):64-72.

3. Data are taken from the largest single controlled study using this dose ($n=266$): *Physicians' Desk Reference.* 54th ed. Montvale, NJ: Medical Economics Company, Inc; 2000:2021-2024.

4. Data taken from Olsson AG, et al. *Clin Ther.* 2001;23:45-61.

5. Data are taken from the EXCEL Study ($n=8245$): Bradford RH, et al. *Arch Intern Med.* 1991;151:43-49.

6. Data are taken from a double-blind trial ($n=138$): Steinhagen-Thiessen E. *Cardiology.* 1994;85:244-254.

7. Data are taken from a double-blind trial ($n=303$): The Lovastatin Pravastatin Study Group. *Am J Cardiol.* 1993;71:810-815.

8. Data are taken as mean from three clinical trials with sample size of at least 500 each (CARE, WOSCOPS, and REGRESS).

9. Data are taken from pooled analysis of two multicenter, double-blind, placebo-controlled studies, $n=277$. Pravachol [package insert]. Princeton, NJ: Bristol-Myers Squibb Co.; 2001.

10. Data are taken from Jones PH, et al. *Am J Cardiol.* 2003;92:152-160.

11. Data are taken from Schneck EW, et al. *Am J Cardiol.* 2003;91:33-41.

12. Data are taken from (1) Farmer JA, et al. *Clin Ther.* 1992;14:708-717; (2) Douste-Blazy P, et al. *Drug Invest.* 1993;6:353-361; (3) Steinhagen-Thiessen E. *Cardiology.* 1994;85:244-254; and (4) Lambrecht LJ, Malini PL. *Acta Cardiol.* 1993;48:541-554.

13. Data are taken from Stein EA, et al. *Am J Cardiol.* 1998;82:311-316.

Heart Protection Study Collaborative Group. MRC/BHF Heart Protection Study of cholesterol lowering with simvastatin in 20,536 high-risk individuals: a randomised placebo-controlled trial. *Lancet*. 2002;360:7-22.

Hennekens CH, Hollar D, Eidelman RS, et al. Update for primary healthcare providers: recent statin trials and revised National Cholesterol Education Program III guidelines. *Med Gen Med*. 2006;8:54.

Keech A, Simes RJ, Barter P, et al; FIELD study investigators. Effects of long-term fenofibrate therapy on cardiovascular events in 9795 people with type 2 diabetes mellitus (the FIELD study): randomised controlled trial. *Lancet*. 2005;366:1849-1861.

Nissen SE, Nicholls SJ, Sipahi I, et al; ASTEROID Investigators. Effect of very high-intensity statin therapy on regression of coronary atherosclerosis: the ASTEROID trial. *JAMA*. 2006;295:1556-1565.

Ridker PM, Danielson E, Fonseca FA, et al; for the JUPITER Study Group. Rosuvastatin to prevent vascular events in men and women with elevated C-reactive protein. *N Engl J Med*. 2008;359:2195-2207.

Rubins HB, Robins SJ, Collins D, et al. Gemfibrozil for the secondary prevention of coronary heart disease in men with low levels of high-density lipoprotein cholesterol. Veterans Affairs High-Density Lipoprotein Cholesterol Intervention Trial Study Group. *N Engl J Med*. 1999;341:410-418.

Sacks FM for the Expert Group on HDL Cholesterol. The role of high-density lipoprotein (HDL) cholesterol in the prevention and treatment of coronary heart disease: expert group recommendations. *Am J Cardiol*. 2002;90:139-143.

Saito I, Folsom AR, Brancati FL, Duncan BB, Chambless LE, McGovern PG. Nontraditional risk factors for coronary heart disease incidence among persons with diabetes: the Atherosclerosis Risk in Communities (ARIC) study. *Ann Intern Med*. 2000;133:81-91.

9

Antiplatelet Therapy and Diabetes: Cardiovascular Risk Reduction

Because of the high risk of CVD in type 2 diabetics, most of these patients (especially in men) should receive aspirin if tolerated. According to an analysis by the Antiplatelet Trialists Collaboration, aspirin lowers the risk for MI and appears to be effective for the secondary prevention of stroke, especially in men. The major issue relates to dosing. In diabetes, there is markedly increased platelet aggregation/adhesion, endothelial cell adhesive properties, and vascular inflammation that likely require an aspirin dosage >81 mg daily. A recent meta-analysis suggests aspirin may not produce a significant reduction of MIs in diabetic women.

The ADA has issued guidelines for aspirin and antiplatelet therapy in adults with diabetes (**Table 9.1**). The ADA recommends that in diabetic patients without specific contraindications, aspirin should be given for:

- Secondary prevention of CV events in both women and men with clinical evidence of macrovascular disease (stroke, transient ischemic attacks, MI, vascular bypass procedures)
- Primary prevention in adult diabetics who have one or more risk factors for CVD (hypertension, smoking, family history of CHD, obesity, dyslipidemia, or albuminuria) or are ≥30 years of age; in other words, in a large majority of diabetic patients.

The ADA indicates that the prophylactic use of aspirin has not been systemically studied in persons <30 years of age and that aspirin should not be recommended for those <21 years of age because of the risk of Reye's syndrome. Doses of enteric-coated aspirin 81 to 325 mg have been recommended. Contraindications cited by the ADA include:

TABLE 9.1 — Recommendations for Use of Antiplatelet Agents in Adults With Diabetes

- Use aspirin therapy (75-162 mg/d) as a primary prevention strategy in those with type 1 or type 2 diabetes at increased CV risk, including those who are >40 yo or who have additional risk factors (eg, family history of CVD, hypertension, smoking, dyslipidemia, or albuminuria)
- Use aspirin therapy (75-162 mg/d) as a secondary prevention strategy in those with diabetes with a history of CVD
- For patients with CVD and documented aspirin allergy, clopidogrel (75 mg/d) should be used
- Combination therapy with aspirin (75-162 mg/d) and clopidogrel (75 mg/d) is reasonable for up to a year after an acute coronary syndrome
- Aspirin therapy is not recommended in people <30 yo, due to lack of evidence of benefit, and is contraindicated in patients <21 yo because of the associated risk of Reye's syndrome

American Diabetes Association. *Diabetes Care.* 2009;32(suppl 1):S13-S61.

- Allergies to aspirin
- Recent gastrointestinal (GI) bleeding
- Clinically active liver disease
- A known propensity to bleed.

The evidence supporting prophylactic aspirin use in adult diabetics is substantial. Three prospective trials in both men and women with diabetes, the Early Treatment Diabetic Retinopathy Study (ETDRS), the HOT study, and the HOPE study, showed benefits of aspirin therapy in the primary prevention of CVD, including MI. The HOT study results also reduced concerns about cerebrovascular bleeding as a complication of aspirin therapy. In patients in the HOT study whose hypertension was controlled, the use of aspirin decreased the occurrence of MI. Although there is considerable evidence supporting the benefits of aspirin in primary prevention in diabetic patients, many diabetics may still not be taking aspirin despite the release of the ADA recommendations and the results of recent trials. Data from a recent meta-analysis which suggest a lack of benefit from aspirin in diabetic women should be clarified when two controlled studies regarding the use of aspirin for primary prevention of CVD in diabetics are reported.

Although a number of antiplatelet agents are currently available, the preponderance of evidence suggests aspirin remains the most effective and least expensive platelet inhibitor. Beneficial effects of aspirin have been demonstrated in patients with diabetes, hypertension, and hypercholesterolemia as well as in people with evidence of CVD. It is unclear at present what is the lowest effective dose of aspirin in diabetic patients, but doses of 160 to 325 mg are most commonly recommended. These doses of aspirin, which are higher than the 81 mg/day recommended for the prevention of CV events in nondiabetics, may be required to counteract the enhanced endothelial adhesiveness and enhanced inflammation that occur in the vasculature of diabetic patients.

There are several new treatments that target platelet activity by inhibiting platelet adhesion and/or aggregation. Aspirin inhibits thromboxane A_2-mediated platelet adhesion. Two other agents, clopidogrel (Plavix) and ticlopidine (Ticlid), have an alternative mechanism of action; they block complementary pathways of platelet activation and aggregation. The different modes of action of these agents and aspirin provide the rationale for combination therapy. Antagonists to the platelet GPIIb/IIIA receptor can prevent fibrinogen binding and block the changes the receptor undergoes to enable it to mediate platelet aggregation. For diabetic patients who cannot tolerate aspirin, ticlopidine and clopidogrel may be used. They are relatively expensive but are otherwise reasonable alternative antiplatelet agents in diabetic patients.

9

American Diabetes Association. Aspirin therapy in diabetes. *Diabetes Care*. 2004;27(suppl 1):S72-S74.

Antiplatelet Trialists' Collaboration. Collaborative overview of random trials with antiplatelet therapy—I: Prevention of death, myocardial infarction, and stroke by prolonged antiplatelet therapy in various categories of patients. *BMJ*. 1994;308:81-106.

De Berardis G, Sacco M, Strippoli GF, et al. Aspirin for primary prevention of cardiovascular events in people with diabetes: meta-analysis of randomised controlled trials. *BMJ*. 2009;339:b4531.

Hart RG, Halperin JL, McBride R, Benavente O, Man-Son-Hing M, Kronmal RA. Aspirin for the primary prevention of stroke and other major vascular events: meta-analysis and hypothesis. *Arch Neurol*. 2000;57:326-332.

Rolka DB, Fagot-Campagna A, Narayan KM. Aspirin use among adults with diabetes: estimates from the Third National Health and Nutrition Examination Survey. *Diabetes Care*. 2001;24:197-201.

10

Control of Diabetes:
Cardiovascular Risk Reduction

Diabetes is an increasingly common disease that may result in disabilities that decrease the quality of life and increase direct and indirect medical costs. Chronic complications accounted for >50% of the estimated $350 billion spent for care of patients with diabetes in the United States. Complications can be significantly reduced by aggressive treatment of risk factors such as hypertension and dyslipidemia in addition to hyperglycemia. Despite this knowledge, the level of care for people with diabetes is suboptimal, even in developed nations. Unfortunately, health policy makers and providers are frequently unaware of (or have failed to act upon) the considerable evidence supporting the role of lifestyle changes (ie, increase in physical activity and adhering to a healthy diet) in the primary prevention of type 2 diabetes and the specific medical therapeutic strategies to prevent or delay the complications of diabetes.

In both patients with type 1 and type 2 diabetes, prospective studies have shown an association between the degree of hyperglycemia and increased risk of microvascular complications (ie, retinopathy, nephropathy), macrovascular events, MI, stroke, peripheral vascular disease, and all-cause mortality. The RR of MI seems to increase with any increase in glycemia to levels >100 mg/dL, whereas the risk for microvascular disease is thought to occur only with more extreme hyperglycemia. The Diabetes Control and Complications Trial (DCCT) showed an association between blood glucose levels and the progression of microvascular complications in patients with type 1 diabetes for HbA_{1C} over the range of 6% to 11% after a mean of 6 years of follow-up. In the UKPDS, a similar relationship was seen in patients with type 2 diabetes. Any reduction in HbA_{1C} reduced the risk of complications, with the lowest risk being in those with HbA_{1C} values in the normal range (<6.0%). However, it should be noted that the CVD benefits of treating hyperglycemia to target values below an HbA_{1C} of 7% have not been proven. The notion that lowering HbA_{1C} levels to <6.0% will reduce CVD morbidity and mortality is currently being tested in the NIH-sponsored ACCORD trial. This study is also testing the hypothesis that lowering the systolic BP to 120 mm Hg may be beneficial in reducing CVD events in persons with type 2 diabetes. The results will probably not be public until 2009. Currently acceptable ranges and goals are given in **Table 10.1**.

Glycation refers to a linkage of carbohydrate to protein. This is an irreversible process in which glucose in the plasma attaches itself to the hemoglobin component of red blood cells. The life span of a red blood cell is 120 days. Therefore, glycated hemoglobin assays, one of which measures HbA_{1C}, reflect the average blood glucose concentration over this period of time. HbA_{1C} measurement depends on the percentage of hemoglobin molecules that have glucose attached (ie, about 5% is average) in non-dysglycemic individuals.

Prevention of Type 2 Diabetes: Lifestyle and Drugs

Observational and interventional studies have shown that lifestyle intervention reduces the risk of developing type 2 DM. In a Swedish study in subjects with an increased risk for development of type 2 diabetes, lifestyle interventions decreased the development of diabetes over 5 years to 10.6% compared with 28.6% in a control group. Improvement in glucose tolerance and decreases in development of type 2 diabetes were related both to increased exercise and weight reduction; both contributed equally and independently to reduction in risk of diabetes.

Several other studies comparing diet, exercise, and diet plus exercise with a nontreatment control group have reported that lifestyle approaches have reduced the occurrence of diabetes by 30% to 55% compared with control groups. The Diabetes Prevention Program (DPP) reported a 56% reduction in NOD with carefully supervised lifestyle interventions in a population at high risk for development of this disease. In contrast, persons randomized to metformin treatment only had a 31%

reduction in development of diabetes. This was a costly study and may not be practical given the increasing limitation of health care resources and poor reimbursement for preventive health care measures. It does, however, emphasize the importance of lifestyle modifications and what can be accomplished.

■ Diet

Dietary treatment is an essential component of management in patients with diabetes. The goals of nutritional intervention in patients with type 2 diabetes are to:

- Maintain near normal or normal blood glucose levels
- Attain and maintain a body weight as close to ideal body weight as possible
- Utilize a low-fat, high-fiber, low-sodium diet that promotes lipid and BP lowering.

Traditional dietary recommendations emphasize reduction of both the total and saturated fat content and replacement with complex carbohydrates (ie, 50% to 55% of dietary calories). However, it must be kept in mind that in type 2 diabetic patients such diets may cause postprandial hyperglycemia. This can be moderated by smaller feedings and increased dietary fiber intake. Generally, a weight-reduction, low-saturated fat diet is appropriate for type 2 diabetics as these patients are at high risk for CVD.

General guidelines for nutritional approaches to patients with diabetes have been developed that take into consideration the heterogeneity of patients with type 2 diabetes (**Table 10.2**). The dietary approach should be monitored not only on the basis of body weight, but also on the impact on metabolic parameters, BP, and the quality of life. In general, this type of diet can be tolerated without difficulty and should include nutritional foods and foods that are high in calcium, potassium, and magnesium.

More than 75% of people with type 2 diabetes are obese; their weight loss is a primary intervention goal. Caloric restriction improves glucose control and the loss of as little as 5% of body weight improves insulin sensitivity, reduces insulin secretion, and decreases

10

TABLE 10.1 — Summary of Glycemic and Lipid Recommendations for Non-pregnant Adults With Diabetes

Glycemic Control

A1C	<7.0%[a]
Preprandial capillary plasma glucose	70-130 mg/dL (3.9-7.2 mmol/L)
Peak postprandial capillary plasma glucose[a]	<180 mg/dL (<10.0 mmol/L)
BP	<130/80 mm Hg

Lipids[b]

LDL	<100 mg/dL (<2.6 mmol/L)
Triglycerides	<150 mg/dL (<1.7 mmol/L)
HDL	>40 mg/dL (>1.0 mmol/L)[c]

Key Concepts in Setting Glycemic Goals

- A1C is the primary target for glycemic control
- Goals should be individualized based on:
  - Duration of diabetes
  - Age/life expectancy
  - Comorbid conditions
  - Known CVD or advanced microvascular complications
  - Hypoglycemia unawareness
  - Individual patient considerations

- More or less stringent glycemic goals may be appropriate for individual patients
- Postprandial glucose may be targeted if A1C goals are not met despite reaching preprandial glucose goals

---

[a] Referenced to a nondiabetic range of 4% to 6% using a Diabetes Control and Complications Trial–based assay. Postprandial glucose measurements should be made 1 to 2 hours after the beginning of a meal, when generally peak levels occur in patients with diabetes.

[b] Current NCEP/ATP III guidelines suggest that in patients with triglycerides ≥200 mg/dL, the "non-HDL cholesterol" (total cholesterol minus HDL) be utilized. The goal is ≤130 mg/dL.

[c] For women, it has been suggested that the HDL goal be increased by 10 mg/dL.

Adapted from: American Diabetes Association. *Diabetes Care.* 2009;32(suppl 1):S13-S61.

TABLE 10.2 — Nutrition Goals, Principles, and Recommendations[a]

- Calories—Sufficient to attain and/or maintain a reasonable body weight for adults, normal growth and development for children and adolescents, and adequate nutrition through pregnancy and lactation
- Protein:
  - 10% to 20% of daily calories
  - No more than adult RDA (0.8 g/kg body weight per day) with evidence of nephropathy (ie, if 2000 calories/d, about 200-400 calories/d of protein; since 1 g protein = 4 calories, then about 50 g = 200 calories/d of protein)
- Fat:
  - Saturated fat <7% to 10% (or about 140-200 calories/d of fat on a 2000 calories/d diet (1 g fat = 9 calories); 15-22 g of fat per day (ie, $9 \times 20 = 180$ calories/d)
  - Polyunsaturated fat up to 10% of total calories (about 200 calories/d on a 2000 calories/d diet)
  - Total fat varies with treatment goals; generally <25% of total calories
  - Predominantly monounsaturated fat
- Cholesterol <250 mg/d
- Carbohydrate:
  - Difference after protein and fat goals have been met
  - Percentage varies with treatment goals
- Sweeteners:
  - Sucrose (ie, table sugar [cane or beet]) need not be restricted; must be substituted as carbohydrate
  - Nutritive sweeteners have no advantage over sucrose and must be substituted as carbohydrate
  - Nonnutritive sweeteners (ie, saccharin, aspartame, acesulfame potassium, and sucralose) approved by the FDA are safe to consume
- Fiber 20-35 g/d (All-Bran, rye bread, etc)
- Sodium <2400 mg/d
- Alcohol—moderate usage, ie, less than two alcoholic beverages daily
- Vitamins and minerals—same as the general population

Goals must always be individualized.

[a] It is important to check food labels for exact amount of each component.

hepatic glucose production. Weight reduction is best accomplished by a combination of caloric restriction and physical activity. Initial or sustained weight reduction is difficult without some increase in physical activity. Increased aerobic activity, in turn, has a direct beneficial effect on insulin sensitivity/glucose utilization and may also lower BP and increase HDL cholesterol levels.

An approach to weight reduction should be realistic, with weight loss of ½ to 1 lb/week recommended. Generally, a decrease of 500 calories/day or 3500 calories/week is needed to produce a loss of 1 lb/week. Substantial weight loss is difficult and many patients will fail to lose weight and keep it down on the first or second try. Having diabetes should be a motivating factor. All patients should be advised to avoid fad diets (ie, diets of the month, high-fat, or high-protein miracle diets). These may work for a short period of time but have not been shown to produce long-term weight loss. The low-carb diet fad has led to dramatic changes in the eating habits of millions of Americans. There is little doubt that such diets will result in weight loss because they basically lower calorie intake. The weight loss over the first week is accounted for mainly by a loss of fluid. The long-term safety of these diets is questionable, as are the long-term very low-carbohydrate, high-protein diets.

If the first miracle diet had worked, there would be no need for a new one every 3 to 6 months. Getting the diabetic patient on a sensible regimen for weight loss is an important step in management and, at the present time, the guidelines noted in **Table 10.2** seem reasonable. More detailed information about diet and diabetes can be found in the numerous publications of the ADA or in standard textbooks on diabetes (see *Chapter 7* regarding guidelines for weight reduction, ideal weights, etc).

10

■ **Exercise**

Both obesity and inactivity contribute significantly to the development of type 2 diabetes. Regular aerobic exercise may delay or prevent type 2 diabetes, and it also helps in therapy of patients with diabetes. Regular aerobic exercise in type 2 diabetic patients helps to:

• Enhance a weight-reduction program
• Improve glycemic control

- Reduce BP and improve the lipid profile
- Enhance quality of life and psychological well-being
- Reduce the requirements for oral antidiabetic agents or insulin.

Exercise, particularly the aerobic variety that includes walking or motion exercise, is beneficial in type 2 diabetes as it helps in maintenance of weight reduction and improves insulin sensitivity. Mechanisms by which aerobic exercise improves insulin sensitivity include decreases in intra-abdominal fat, increases in insulin-sensitive skeletal muscle fibers, and reduction in FFAs that interfere with insulin action. In addition, exercise provides the additional benefits of possibly lowering BP, improving CV function, raising HDL, and lowering triglycerides.

There are several caveats that should be considered in recommending exercise in type 2 diabetic patients. Because many type 2 patients are obese and have led sedentary lives, they are often in poor physical condition. A thorough history and physical examination and an electrocardiogram should generally be performed before these patients engage in exercise. Lower levels of exercise should be initiated and resistance training (ie, weight lifting) should be done with caution (lifting of 5- to 10-lb weights can probably be undertaken without concern). If an individual does plan to engage in heavier weight lifting or vigorous exercise (ie, running), he or she should probably have an exercise stress test and a careful ophthalmologic examination to avoid exacerbation of retinopathy. Strenuous exercise is contraindicated in diabetic patients with active proliferative retinopathy, significant neuropathy, or CVD. Peripheral neuropathy involving decreased sensitivity in the soles of the feet and inadequate peripheral pulses preclude running or jogging. In diabetics who exercise, it is important that they have comfortable shoes with appropriate arch supports. Appropriate precautions for diabetic patients with medical complications are given in **Table 10.3**.

Most diabetic patients can undertake a program of walking. Biking and swimming are usually safe and

TABLE 10.3 — Precautions for Diabetic Patients With Medical Complications

- Insensitive feet or peripheral vascular insufficiency:
  - Avoid running
  - Choose walking, cycling, or swimming
  - Emphasize proper footwear
- Untreated or recently treated proliferative retinopathy; avoid exercises associated with:
  - Increased intra-abdominal pressure (ie, heavy weight lifting)
  - Valsalvalike maneuvers
  - Rapid head movements
  - Possible eye trauma
- Hypertension:
  - Avoid heavy lifting
  - Avoid Valsalvalike maneuvers

useful exercises in patients with neuropathy where foot placement and gait may be compromised. Generally, diabetic persons should begin slowly, exercise at regular intervals at least 3 to 4 times a week, and gradually increase the duration and intensity of their exercise program. Flexibility stretching is important to promote range of motion and prevent muscle and joint injury; this is especially important in the elderly diabetic. There is no reason why diabetic patients cannot participate in sports such as golf or tennis. Limitations should include chest or leg pain (intermittent claudication). Finally, armchair exercises can be performed by those patients confined to a wheelchair or those with very limited mobility. A diet and exercise program is useful not only in helping with glucose control but also may favorably impact lipid and BP abnormalities.

One potential problem associated with any aerobic exercise program is hypoglycemia in patients receiving oral antidiabetic agents or insulin. Hypoglycemia can occur during or as long as 12 hours after aerobic exercise. Monitoring of blood glucose is useful in adjusting oral medications or insulin to prevent exercise-induced hypoglycemia. Timing of exercise is important in the diabetic patient. Exercise performed between 3 PM and 5 PM may reduce nighttime hepatic glucose production and thus decrease fasting blood glucose levels. In addition, exercise after eating may reduce the postprandial hyperglycemia that often occurs in type 2 diabetes and which is increasingly associated with microvascular and macrovascular complications. The benefits of aerobic exercise in type 2 diabetic patients are achieved with exercise at least 3 times per week or every other day. Weight reduction is enhanced by exercise sessions carried out 5 to 6 times weekly (**Table 10.4**).

TABLE 10.4 — Guidelines for Safe Exercise and Insulin Use

- At all times, patients should carry an identification card and wear a bracelet, necklace, or tag that identifies them as having diabetes
- If insulin is used:
  - Avoid exercise during peak insulin action
  - Administer insulin away from working limbs
- If the patient takes a single daily dose of intermediate-acting insulin, decrease the dose by as much as 30% to 35% before exercise
- If a combination of short- and intermediate-acting insulin is being given, decrease or omit the short-acting insulin by up to one third on days when exercise is planned. This may produce hyperglycemia later in the day that requires a second injection of short-acting insulin
- If only short-acting insulin is being used, reduce the preexercise dose and reduce the postexercise dose based on self-monitoring of blood glucose. The total dose may need to be reduced by as much as 30% to 50% on days when exercise is planned
- Be alert for signs of hypoglycemia during and for several hours after exercise. Have immediate access to a source of readily absorbable carbohydrate (such as glucose tablets) to treat hypoglycemia
- Take sufficient fluids before, after, and if necessary, during exercise to prevent dehydration

Diabetic Retinopathy

The importance of regular ophthalmologic evaluations and early detection and treatment of visual problems in diabetic persons cannot be overemphasized. More than 5000 cases of blindness related to diabetes occur in the

United States yearly. Diabetes is the leading cause of new blindness in Americans between the ages of 20 and 74 years. Hypertension (and probably hyperlipidemia) accelerates the development of diabetic retinopathy. More than 60% of patients with type 2 diabetes have some form of diabetic retinopathy within 20 years after the diagnosis is made. Loss of vision associated with proliferative retinopathy and macular edema can be reduced by 50% with laser photocoagulation if identified in time.

This is the therapy of choice in patients who have developed proliferative retinopathy; it reduces the risk of sudden and/or severe visual loss by up to 60%. The intent of photocoagulation is to stop neovascularization before recurrent hemorrhages into the vitreous cause irreversible visual loss. On occasions when retinal detachment and massive vitreous hemorrhage occur, closed vitrectomy can be performed to remove blood vitreous and fibrous tissue. In at least half of the cases, vision can be restored by this procedure.

Diabetic retinopathy, either in the form of macular edema or proliferative retinopathy, does not typically cause visual problems until a relatively advanced stage has been reached. Control of metabolic abnormalities and BP is important in the prevention and lessening of progression of both background (nonproliferative) and proliferative retinopathy. Therefore, early management results are better when the disease is diagnosed early and, accordingly, a yearly ophthalmologic examination by an ophthalmologist or optometrist experienced in diagnosing diabetic retinopathy is important.

Prevention of Lower Extremity Peripheral Vascular Complications

More than 50% of nontraumatic amputations in the United States occur in diabetics, and it has been estimated that more than half of these amputations could have been prevented with proper foot care, control of abnormal glucose metabolism, hyperlipidemia, and BP in people who are hypertensive. Foot lesions leading to nontraumatic amputations are the result of peripheral vascular disease, polyneuropathy, and superimposed infections. The sudden development of a painful foot or ankle lesion, usually secondary to some trauma or irritation, often indicates that there is underlying vascular disease, which is clinically indicated by decreased or absent pulses, dependent rubor, and pallor on leg elevation (**Table 10.5**). The degree of vascular disease and its potential for treatment by surgical intervention can be determined by Doppler ultrasonography followed up with angiography. Revascularization procedures, such as bypass or angioplasty, may be helpful in treating patients for nonhealing lesions, claudication, or the healing of amputation suture/incision sites. On the other hand, these procedures are sometimes ineffective because of the diffuse nature of vascular lesions in diabetic patients. Smoking cessation is extremely important in the prevention of peripheral vascular disease and its progression in diabetic persons. Proper foot care and measures to slow down vascular injury (ie, glycemic control, management of lipids, platelet disorders, and normalization of BP) are important and, in many cases, effective in preventing peripheral vascular disease in diabetics.

Pharmacologic Therapy

Pharmacologic therapy should be instituted in conjunction with diet and exercise. Agents currently available for type 2 diabetics if dietary and exercise programs are ineffective in reducing blood glucose and HbA_{1C} levels to a normal range include sulfonylureas and related compounds, biguanides, thiazolidinediones, α-glucosidase inhibitors, dipeptidyl peptidase IV (DPP-IV) inhibitors, exenatide, and insulin. **Table 10.6** lists the available oral antidiabetic agents. A rational approach to using available agents involves using those drugs particularly suited to the stage and extent of the disease and progressing to combination therapy, which is eventually necessary in most patients (**Figure 10.1**).

■ **Agents That Enhance Insulin Secretion**
Sulfonylureas

Sulfonylureas, such as tolbutamide (Orinase) and tolazamide (Tolinase), and the newer preparations, such

TABLE 10.5 — Warning Symptoms and Signs of Diabetic Foot Problems

Cause	Symptoms	Signs
Vascular	Cold feet; intermittent claudication involving calf or foot; pain at rest, especially nocturnal, relieved by dependency	Absent pedal, popliteal, or femoral pulses; femoral bruits; dependent rubor; plantar pallor on elevation; prolonged capillary filling time (>3-4 sec); decreased skin temperature
Neurologic	*Sensory:* burning, tingling, or crawling sensations; pain and hypersensitivity; cold feet *Motor:* weakness (foot drop) *Autonomic:* diminished sweating	*Sensory:* deficits (vibratory, then pain and temperature perception), hyperesthesia *Motor:* diminished to absent deep tendon reflexes (↓ Achilles, then patellar reflexes); weakness *Autonomic:* diminished-to-absent sweating
Musculoskeletal	Gradual changes in foot shape, sudden painless change in foot shape, with swelling, without history of trauma	Cavus feet with claw toes; drop foot; "rocker-bottom" foot (Charcot's joint); neuropathic arthropathy
Dermatologic	Painful wounds; slow-healing or nonhealing wounds or necrosis; skin color changes (cyanosis, redness); chronic scaling, itching, or dry feet; recurrent infections (paronychia, athlete's foot)	*Skin:* abnormal dryness; chronic tinea infections; keratotic lesions with or without hemorrhage (plantar or digital); trophic ulcer *Hair:* diminished or absent *Nails:* trophic changes; onychomycosis; sublingual ulceration or abscess; ingrown nails with paronychia

10

TABLE 10.6 — Characteristics of Currently Available Oral Antidiabetic Agents

Generic Name	Trade Name	Recommended Starting Dose (mg)	Recommended Daily Maximum Dose (mg)	Dose Frequency
***Sulfonylureas*[a]**				
First Generation				
Acetohexamide	Dymelor	125 bid	1500	bid
Chlorpropamide	Diabinese	250 qd	500	qd
Tolazamide	Tolinase	100 qd	1000	bid
Tolbutamide	Orinase	250 bid	3000	tid
Second Generation				
Glimepiride	Amaryl	1-2 qd	8	qd
Glipizide	Glucotrol	5 qd	40	bid
Glipizide (extended release)	Glucotrol XL	5 qd	20	qd
Glyburide	DiaBeta, Micronase	2.5-5 qd	20	bid
	Glynase PresTab	1.5-3 qd	12	bid
Glinides				
Repaglinide[b]	Prandin	0.5 bid-qid w/meals	4	bid-qid w/meals
Nateglinide[c]	Starlix	120 tid w/meals	360	bid-qid w/meals
Glinide/Biguanide Combination Agent				
Repaglinide/metformin	Prandimet	1/500	10/2500	bid-qid w/meals

Thiazolidinediones[c]			
Pioglitazone	Actos	15-30 qd	qd
Rosiglitazone	Avandia	4 qd or 2 bid	bid-qd
Biguanide[d]			
Metformin	Glucophage	500 qd with evening meal	bid-tid
	Fortamet	500-1000 qd	qd
	Glucophage XR	500 qd	qd
	Glumetza	1000 qd	qd
Alpha-Glucosidase Inhibitors[d]			
Acarbose	Precose	25 tid w/meals	bid-tid w/meals
Miglitol	Glyset	25 tid w/meals	bid-tid w/meals
DPP-IV Inhibitor			
Sitagliptin	Januvia	100	qd with or without meals
Sulfonylurea/Biguanide Combination Agents			
Glipizide/metformin	Metaglip	2.5/250 qd w/meals	bid w/meals
Glyburide/metformin	Glucovance	1.25/250 qd w/meals	bid w/meals

Continued

10

225

TABLE 10.6 — *Continued*

Generic Name	Trade Name	Recommended Starting Dose (mg)	Recommended Daily Maximum Dose (mg)	Dose Frequency
Thiazolidinedione/Biguanide Combination Agents				
Pioglitazone/metformin	Actoplus Met	15/500 or 15/850 w/meals	45/2550	bid w/meals
Rosiglitazone/metformin	Avandamet	2/500 bid w/meals	8/2000	bid w/meals
Thiazolidinedione/Sulfonylurea Combination Agents				
Pioglitazone/glimepiride	Duetact	30/2 or 30/4	45/8	qd
Rosiglitazone/glimepiride	Avandaryl	4/1 or 4/2	8/4	qd
DPP-IV Inhibitor/Biguanide Combination Agent				
Sitagliptin/metformin	Janumet	50/500	100/2000	bid w/meals
Bile Acid Sequestrant				
Colesevelam	Welchol	3750 mg	3750 mg	bid-qd

[a] Starting dose for elderly and lean adults with diabetes may need to be reduced by up to 50%.
[b] Selection of initial dose depends on the patient's glucose level.
[c] Starting dose may be reduced by 50% when patients are near the A1C goal.
[d] The dose of metformin, acarbose, and miglitol must be titrated slowly to limit gastrointestinal side effects.

Modified from: *Physicians' Desk Reference 2009.* 63rd ed. Montvale, NJ: Thomson PDR; 2008.

as glipizide (Glucotrol, Glucotrol XL) and glimepiride (Amaryl), were the first of the oral hypoglycemic agents. Their primary action is to enhance insulin secretion. Because they can increase insulin secretion at all glucose levels, they may cause hypoglycemia. All sulfonylureas bind to the β-cell of the pancreas and close ATP-sensitive potassium channels. As a result, calcium channels open, leading to an increase in cytoplasmic calcium, thus stimulating insulin secretion. One of these agents, glimepiride (Amaryl), appears to exert relatively selective inhibition of the ATP-sensitive potassium channel on the β-cell of the pancreas, having little or no effect on the vascular or cardiac ATP-sensitive potassium channels. This means that this agent may not impair preischemic reconditioning in the heart.

To a lesser extent than for insulin therapy, sulfonylureas, through resultant hyperinsulinemia, may cause weight gain as well as development of hypoglycemia. Some data suggests that the use of long-acting glipizide (Glucotrol XL) may result in less weight gain and, in addition, offers sustained glucose control over 24 hours. The kidney is important in the clearance of most sulfonylureas. Therefore, these agents should be used with caution in persons with impaired renal function. Sulfonylureas should also be used with caution in persons with impaired liver function. The concern that sulfonylureas directly increase CVD mortality (a concern originally raised by the University Group Diabetes Project) has been largely allayed by the UKPDS. The UKPDS demonstrated that in the presence of a comparable degree of glycemic control, mortality did not differ in patients treated with either insulin or sulfonylureas. Sulfonylureas are generally appropriate drugs in patients with relative insulin deficiency. Such patients would typically be lean, with lower basal and postprandial insulin levels. In addition, based on the UKPDS, these patients tend to be younger (<46 years of age) and more likely to require insulin. Dosage and frequency of administration are listed in **Table 10**.6.

Repaglinide (Prandin)

Repaglinide is a nonsulfonylurea secretagogue of the meglitinide class. It binds to a nonsulfonylurea β-cell

FIGURE 10.1 — Treatment Algorithm for Pharmacologic Therapy for Type 2 Diabetes

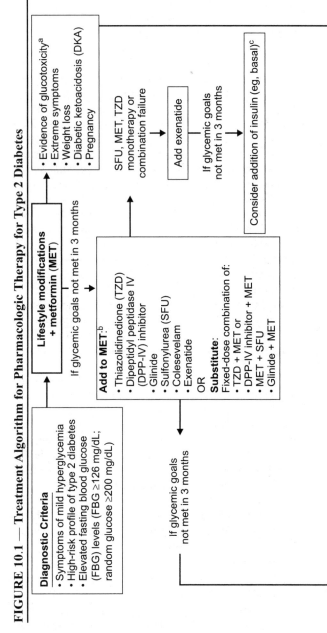

228

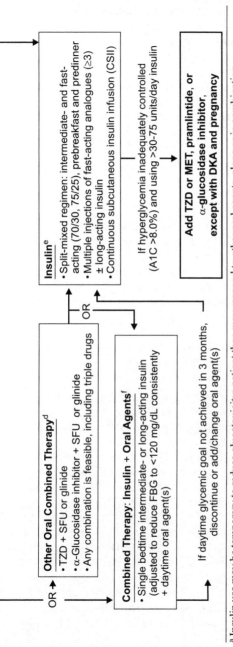

Other Oral Combined Therapy[d]

- TZD + SFU or glinide
- α-Glucosidase inhibitor + SFU or glinide
- Any combination is feasible, including triple drugs

OR →

Combined Therapy: Insulin + Oral Agents[f]

- Single bedtime intermediate- or long-acting insulin (adjusted to reduce FBG to <120 mg/dL consistently + daytime oral agent(s)

If daytime glycemic goal not achieved in 3 months, discontinue or add/change oral agent(s)

OR

Insulin[e]

- Split-mixed regimen: intermediate- and fast-acting (70/30, 75/25), prebreakfast and predinner
- Multiple injections of fast-acting analogues (≥3) ± long-acting insulin
- Continuous subcutaneous insulin infusion (CSII)

If hyperglycemia inadequately controlled (A1C >8.0%) and using >30–75 units/day insulin

Add TZD or MET, pramlintide, or α-glucosidase inhibitor, except with DKA and pregnancy

---

[a] Insulin use may be temporary to reduce glucotoxicity: patient then may respond to other oral agents, alone or in combination.

[b] Choice of therapy depends on individual patient characteristics.

[c] Not an FDA-approved combination.

[d] Some combinations not yet Food and Drug Administration (FDA)-approved indications.

[e] Choice of insulin regimen based on individual assessment.

[f] For patient selection of combination therapy, see discussion in text.

10

receptor and stimulates insulin secretion by inhibiting the ATP-sensitive potassium channel. It has rapid onset and offset of action and, therefore, needs to be taken with meals. It decreases the postprandial glycemic increase and may cause less weight gain and hypoglycemia than sulfonylureas. Repaglinide is primarily excreted in the feces, with little or no excretion by the kidney. Therefore, it can be used in individuals with impaired renal function. Since it is metabolized by the liver, it should not be used in patients with hepatic dysfunction. As with sulfonylureas, repaglinide shows an added benefit when given with metformin.

Nateglinide (Starlix)

Nateglinide is an N-acetylphenylalanine derivative that acts by inhibiting the same ATP-sensitive potassium channel that is inhibited by sulfonylureas. It also has a rapid onset and offset of action and, therefore, needs to be taken with each meal. Nateglinide, like repaglinide, is metabolized to inactive metabolites by the liver and excreted in the feces. There is little or no excretion by the kidney.

■ Agents That Alter Insulin Action
Metformin (Glucophage)

Glucose lowering by this drug occurs primarily by decreasing hepatic glucose production, and to a lesser extent, by decreasing peripheral insulin resistance. Metformin acts by causing the translocation of glucose transporters from the microsomal fraction to the plasma membrane of hepatic and skeletal muscle cells. It does not stimulate insulin release and does not cause hypoglycemia. Moreover, it does not cause weight gain, and may improve the lipid profile by causing a decline in total and VLDL, triglycerides, total cholesterol, and LDL cholesterol, and an increase in HDL cholesterol. It is best suited for obese patients with type 2 diabetes who are unresponsive to diet alone and who are assumed to be insulin resistant. It has some anorectic properties and causes less weight gain than other oral agents or insulin. It is effective as monotherapy or in combination with other agents, such as insulin or insulin secretagogues, other insulin-sensitizing drugs, or inhibitors of glucose absorption such as acarbose. Results of studies have shown that the addition of nateglinide to metformin improved glycemic control in patients on metformin monotherapy who have failed to achieve HbA_{1C} goals.

The major risk of this drug, lactic acidosis, occurs with a frequency of 1:120,000 patient-year. Its major route of excretion is through the kidneys. Metformin is contraindicated in those with renal disease (creatinine $\geq$1.5 in males; $\geq$1.4 in females), in the presence of hepatic disease, and in patients with tissue ischemia. In addition, the drug should be withheld for 48 hours after intravenous contrast administration. Metformin has advantages of not causing weight gain, not generally causing hypoglycemia, and offering good glucose control because of its inhibition of overnight gluconeogenesis. It is an ideal oral agent for overweight type 2 diabetic patients.

Metformin Combination Formulations

Metformin is now available in fixed-dose combination formulations with five other antidiabetic agents, namely:

- Metformin + the sulfonylurea glyburide (Glucovance)
- Metformin + sulfonylurea glipizide (Metaglip)
- Metformin + the thiazolidinedione rosiglitazone (Avandamet)
- Metformin + the thiazolidinedione pioglitazone (Actoplus Met)
- Metformin + the selective DPP-IV inhibitor sitagliptin (Janumet)

10

Some of these medications have been available for many years; clinical trials have provided substantial evidence that early combination therapy with two different drugs that have different mechanisms of action can provide additional benefits in terms of glucose control. In addition, combination formulations can simplify the multidrug regimens typically used in diabetic patients.

■ Thiazolidinediones (Avandia, Actos)

These drugs appear to act by binding to receptors that influence the differentiation of fibroblasts into adipocytes; free fatty acid levels are lowered. Clinically, their major effect is to decrease insulin resistance; this requires the presence of insulin to exert beneficial effects. In contrast to sulfonylureas and metformin, the effects of the thiazolidinediones may be progressive over time, and their full hypoglycemic effects may not be achieved until after 10 weeks of therapy. An elevated C peptide and being overweight may help to predict a beneficial response to these drugs as well as to metformin. These drugs are also usually synergistic with metformin in improving glucose control. Moreover, as insulin resistance is often accompanied by relative insulin deficiency, either a thiazolidinedione or metformin is often most effective when either or both drugs are given along with insulin or an insulin secretagogue.

The thiazolidinediones approved by the Food and Drug Administation (FDA) are rosiglitazone (Avandia) and pioglitazone (Actos). Both drugs cause some weight gain and increased adiposity. However, the increase in body fat may be associated with a shift from visceral to subcutaneous fat. This class of drugs can cause water retention and hemodilution. Therefore, they are not recommended for use in persons with stage 3 or 4 heart failure, and should be used with caution in anyone with cardiac dysfunction. Since they are metabolized by the liver, they should not be used in patients with hepatic dysfunction. It is recommended that liver enzymes be checked prior to the initiation of therapy with these agents and periodically thereafter.

In summary, both rosiglitazone and pioglitazone:

- Substantially reduce glucose and HbA_{1C} levels
- Reduce insulin resistance
- Cause small reductions in SBP and DBP
- Reduce liver enzyme ALT levels
- Lower FFAs
- Reduce albuminuria
- Reduce markers of inflammation and increase adiponectin levels.

On the other hand, they increase subcutaneous fat and may cause peripheral edema, and increase the risk for heart failure in susceptible populations.

A meta-analysis of data from 42 trials indicated that the use of rosiglitazone resulted in a small but significant increased risk of MI and a small but not statistically significant increased risk of death. Out of a total of 15,560 patients in the rosiglitazone group, there were 86 MIs compared with 72 in the 12,283-patient control group, a difference of 14 events; 39 cardiovascular deaths occurred in the rosiglitazone group compared with 22 in the group not taking rosiglitazone, a difference of 17. The authors excluded six trials that did not report any MIs and CVD-related deaths because of an inability to calculate odds ratios from these studies. Thus it is possible that the exclusion of these studies may have artificially magnified the effects of rosiglitazone on CVD events. Inclusion of these reports may have rendered the odds ratio for rosiglitazone-related events nonsignificant.

Although no prospective CVD trial with rosiglitazone has been completed, a placebo-controlled randomized prospective trial using pioglitazone (PROACTIVE) reported a 10% trend favoring a reduction in total CVD events with pioglitazone compared with placebo. The beneficial trends in events were not present until after 1 year of follow-up, pointing out one of the major limitations in the small trials with rosiglitazone.

An outcome trial using rosiglitazone (RECORD), in which the primary outcome is CVD events should provide more definitive data on the risks and benefits of rosiglitazone on CVD has not been terminated prematurely by the data and safety monitoring committee after 3 years of follow-up. The results of the ongoing RECORD trial may help to further clarify this issue.

Meanwhile, additional data on the effect of rosiglitazone on mortality risk come from the DREAM trial in which 5269 people with IFG or IGT, or both, and no previous CV disease were randomized to receive the ACE inhibitor, ramipril (15 mg/day) or placebo, or rosiglitazone (8 mg/day) or placebo, using a 2×2 factorial design; they were followed for a median of 3 years. The primary outcome was a composite of incident diabetes or death (included since undiagnosed diabetes may be more frequent in people who die than in those who do not). Regression to normal glucose levels at 2 years was a secondary outcome measure. Ramipril modestly improved glycemic status, including a 9% nonsignificant reduction in the incidence of diabetes and a significant 16% increase in regression to normal glucose levels. The results with rosiglitazone were more impressive, namely, 11.6% of patients in the rosiglitazone group compared with 26.0% in the placebo group developed the composite primary outcome (P <0.0001). Of particular note is the fact that the number of deaths was similar in both groups (30 and 33, rosiglitazone and placebo, respectively). Similarly, 10.6% of rosiglitazone-treated patients developed diabetes compared with 25% of those who received placebo (P <0.0001), a risk reduction of 62%. The proportion of patients who became normoglycemic by at least 2 years was significantly greater with rosiglitazone than with placebo (50.5% vs 30.3%, respectively; P <0.0001).

■ Agents That Delay the Absorption of Carbohydrates
Alpha-Glucosidase Inhibitors (Precose, Glyset)

Alpha-glucosidase inhibitors include acarbose (Precose) and miglitol (Glyset). These agents inhibit the enzymatic degradation of sucrose, maltose, and other oligosaccharides. Thus they delay the absorption of carbohydrates and thereby lower the increase in postprandial blood glucose. The glucose-lowering effect of these drugs is proportional to the carbohydrate content of the diet. Both drugs must be taken with meals. Side effects are primarily gastrointestinal. Disaccharides not absorbed in the small intestine as a result of the action of these drugs enter the large intestine, where they are metabolized by bacteria to short-chain fatty acids. This may result in abdominal bloating, flatulence, and diarrhea that may be minimized by slowly titrating the dose of these drugs. Although alpha-glucosidase inhibitors do not cause hypoglycemia when used alone, they may increase the risk of hypoglycemia when combined with insulin or insulin secretagogue therapy such as the sulfonylureas.

Although poorly absorbed, renal impairment can lead to an increase in plasma levels of these medications. Therefore they should not be used in patients with renal impairment. These agents are very useful in patients who are not controlled on several other oral agents. Their GI side effects can be minimized by careful titration of dosing.

■ Insulin

Insulin therapy is indicated in the treatment of all type 1 patients and in type 2 patients for initial therapy of severe hyperglycemia, after failure of oral agents, during perioperative periods, during and following an MI, or other acute hyperglycemic states. Insulin has been used in various combinations in type 2 diabetics, and new insulin analogues are becoming available for clinical use. The first available insulin analogue was lispro insulin, representing a two–amino acid modification of regular insulin. Lispro insulin does not form aggregates following subcutaneous injection, allowing it to have a more rapid onset and a shorter duration of action. These properties may help minimize the postprandial rise in glucose and decrease the risk of late hypoglycemia. Any insulin therapy can, however, result in a weight gain and a tendency to develop hypoglycemia. The results of the UKPDS do not support the notion that exogenous insulin increases the risk of CVD. Insulin is often used in conjunction with sensitizing agents, but this combination can lead to significant weight gain (especially the combination of insulin and thiazolidinediones such as Avandia or Actos). Ultimately, insulin therapy may become necessary in many patients with type 2 diabetes as pancreatic β-cell failure ensues. The addition of bedtime insulin to sulfonylureas and sensitizing agents may delay β-cell failure. Finally, it is appropriate to use insulin therapy during hospitalization for myocardial ischemia, stroke, and perioperative procedures if blood glucose levels are high. It is also important to maintain good glycemic control and avoid hypoglycemia (blood sugar <80-100 mg/dL) during hospitalization.

10

Details regarding types of insulin available and more specific regimens for use can be found in standard books on diabetes.

■ Incretin Hormone Therapy

Research has demonstrated that the intestinal peptides (incretin hormones), glucose-dependent insulinotropic polypeptide and glucagonlike peptide-1 (GLP-1), play an important role in regulating insulin secretion and postprandial glucose levels. In healthy subjects, postprandial levels of GLP-1 rise rapidly after a meal, whereas patients with diabetes or IGT exhibit reduced levels of meal-stimulated circulating GLP-1. Thus the administration of exogenous GLP-1 has the potential to normalize fasting and postprandial plasma glucose levels in patients with type 2 diabetes. Despite these features, the therapeutic potential of GLP-1 has been limited by its rapid and extensive degradation.

Exenatide (Byetta)

Exendin-4 (exenatide) is a naturally occurring incretin mimetic. In mammals, exendin-4 exhibits antidiabetic activities similar to those of native GLP-1 but is resistant to degradation; this contributes to its longer half-life compared with GLP-1.

Exenatide has been approved as adjunctive therapy to improve glycemic control in patients with type 2 DM who are taking metformin, a sulfonylurea, or their combination, but who have not achieved adequate glycemic control (ie, in patients resistant to usual therapy). Exenatide therapy must be given by subcutaneous injection twice daily at any time within the 60-minute period before the morning and evening meals.

A number of clinical trials, several of which were of >1½ years in duration, have demonstrated the efficacy and tolerability of exenatide in combination with one or more antidiabetic agents. Patients in phase 3 trials on the highest dose (10 mcg) of exenatide also showed statistically significant reductions in body weight of approximately 2 kg. Exenatide may be used as an alternative to insulin in patients being treated with metformin and a sulfonylurea.

Sitagliptin (Januvia)

Since incretin hormone actions are rapidly terminated by enzyme DPP-IV, the use of DPP-IV inhibitors offers another strategy for the treatment of patients with type 2 diabetes. One of the advantages of DPP-IV inhibitors is that they can be taken orally.

Sitagliptin, a selective DPP-IV inhibitor, is approved for monotherapy as an adjunct to diet and exercise to improve glycemic control in patients with type 2 diabetes, and in combination with metformin or a thiazolidinedione agonist. In patients with type 2 diabetes, the recommended dose of sitagliptin is 100 mg once daily as monotherapy or as part of combination therapy. Sitagliptin can be taken with or without food. Dosage adjustment is recommended in patients with evidence of renal insufficiency.

Several controlled studies of sitagliptin used as monotherapy or added to another antidiabetic agent have reported that sitagliptin treatment results in significant reductions in HbA_{1C} and improved glucose control (**Figure 10.2**). The DPP-IV inhibitors only exert their effects on the pancreas to increase insulin secretion and lower glucagon secretion in response to elevated blood glucose levels. Thus they are usually not associated with hypoglycemia. They also have the advantage that they are weight neutral.

■ Bile Acid Sequestrant
Colesevelam

Colesevelam (Welchol), non-absorbed polymer that binds bile acids in the intestine thereby impeding their resorption, was recently approved as an adjunct to diet and exercise to improve glycemic control adults with type 2 diabetes. It had been previously approved for treatment of primary hyperlipidemia as monotherapy or in combination with an HMG-A reductase inhibitor (statin).

Use of Mineral Supplements

Certain mineral compounds, such as chromium picolinate, have been found, both in animal and human studies, to increase the effects of insulin in clearing blood glucose

FIGURE 10.2 — Effects of Sitagliptin Added to Ongoing Metformin Therapy on Glycemic Control in Patients With Type 2 Diabetes

A. Mean (SE) A1C Over Time[a]

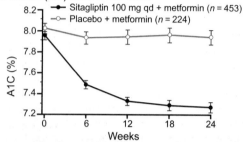

B. Mean (SE) Plasma Glucose Concentration (mg/dL) at Baseline and Week 24 Following Glucose Challenge[b,c]

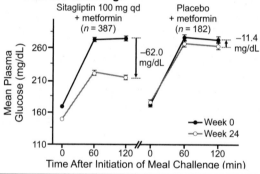

[a] LS mean difference between groups [95% CI] in A1C = −0.65% [−0.77, −0.53]; P <0.001.

[b] Patients ingested a standardized meal consisting of two nutrition bars and one nutrition drink (−680 kcal; carbohydrates, 111 g; fat, 14 g; protein, 26 g.

[c] LS mean difference between groups in change from baseline at week 24 in 2-hour postmeal glucose [95% CI] = −50.6 mg/dL [−60.5, −40.8]; P <0.001.

Modified from: Karasik A, et al. Poster presented at: 66th Scientific Sessions of the American Diabetes Association; June 9-13, 2006; Washington, DC. Poster 501-P.

and increasing glycogen deposition in muscles. A study suggests that this supplement may be helpful in reducing HbA_{1C} in poorly controlled hypertensive diabetics.

Glycemic Control: Does It Reduce Cardiovascular Events?

The DCCT provided unequivocal evidence of substantive reductions in chronic microvascular complications (eg, retinopathy, nephropathy, and neuropathy) in a group of type 1 diabetic patients in whom intensive therapy maintained glucose at near-normal levels over a 6-year period with a mean HbA_{1C} slightly above 7% compared with 9% in controls. The UKPDS also showed a significant risk reduction for microvascular events. However, the results of the UKPDS also demonstrated that rigorous glycemic control was difficult. For example, median HbA_{1C} concentrations 10 years after the study was initiated were higher than baseline values in patients assigned to intensive treatment. This inability to tightly control glucose may have accounted, in part, for the findings of greater benefit of BP lowering compared with tight glucose control. For example, there were substantial reductions in end points related to diabetes (24%), deaths related to diabetes (32%), and microvascular disease (37%) in people achieving tight control of BP. In contrast, improvements in end points with tight glycemic control were not as great: reduction of end points related to diabetes (only 10%), and microvascular disease (25%). There were no significant benefits in either stroke or heart failure reduction in those in the intensive glucose-lowering group compared with a 44% decrease in stroke and a 56% decrease in heart failure in the group assigned to tight BP control (a difference of only $-10/-5$ mm Hg between the tight and less well-controlled group).

The benefits of initially lowered BP were not maintained 10 years after the study ended, suggesting that BP control must be maintained over time. In contrast, the early intensive efforts to lower HbA_{1C} (even if not to target levels) appeared to result in long-term benefit.

A recent meta-analysis of five randomized studies of >30,000 patients with type 2 diabetes reported results of aggressive glucose-lowering regimens which reduced HbA_{1C} by 0.9% more than in patients who received standard therapy. Intensive glycemic control resulted in a significant 17% reduction in events of nonfatal MI (OR 0.83, 95% CI 0.75-0.93), and a 15% reduction in coronary artery disease events (0.85, 0.77-0.93). Intensive glycemic control had no significant effect on stroke (0.93, 0.81-1.06) or all-cause mortality (1.02, 0.87-1.19). Overall, patients with intensive glycemic control compared with those with standard glycemic control significantly reduced coronary events without an increased risk of death.

In the Action to Control Cardiovascular Risk in Diabetes (ACCORD) study, where >10,000 patients with a median glycated hemoglobin level received either intensive therapy with a target of <6% or standard therapy with a target of 7% to 7.9%, no statistically significant difference in outcome was noted despite achieved levels of 6.4% and 7.5% in HbA_{1C} in the intensive-therapy group compared with the standard-therapy group. Hypoglycemia and weight gain were more frequent in the intensive-care group. There were also more deaths in that cohort. Over a 3.5-year period of time, this study concluded that intensive care may actually increase mortality.

In contrast, the Action in Diabetes and Vascular Disease: Preterax and Diamicron Modified Release Control Evaluation (ADVANCE) study reported that intensive care to achieve an HbA_{1C} ≤6.5% (compared with a group with 7.3% HbA_{1C}) resulted in a 10% reduction in major macro- and micro-CV events, largely as a result of a 21% reduction in nephropathy. No significant effects of glucose control were noted on retinopathy or deaths. The study reported an additive effect if two treatment strategies were employed (ie, lowering BP and lowering HbA_{1C} levels), with a significant reduction in risk of 28% for a renal event, 33% reduction in the risk of new or worsening nephropathy, and a 54% reduction in the risk of new-onset microalbuminuria with both strategies compared with a program that did not target lowering BP or lowering glucose levels.

In yet another study, the 5-year Veterans Affairs Diabetes Trial (VADT), the achieved HbA_{1C} levels in the intensive-care group were 6.9% compared with 8.4% in the standard-therapy group. No significant differences between these two groups in CV events, death, or microvascular complications were noted.

These recent studies suggest that there is evidence to suggest that control of blood glucose levels in type 2 diabetics will improve outcome. Intensive care with decreases in HbA_{1C} <7%, however, may not always result in greater benefit than less vigorous approaches. They also indirectly emphasize the importance of control of other risk factors in diabetes, ie, hypertension, obesity, and hyperlipidemia, to achieve reduction of CV events.

Study Results With Antidiabetic Therapy

The overall results of the UKPDS can be subdivided into two components:

- Results in patients randomized to insulin and to sulfonylurea agents (glyburide or chlorpropamide) (n=2729)
- Results achieved in overweight patients randomized to metformin therapy (n=342).

Both treatment cohorts were compared with patients who were treated less intensively initially with diet alone. By the end of the study, however, many patients in the diet-alone group required some form of medication for treatment of hyperglycemia. Findings from the sulfonylurea and/or insulin arm of the study showed that the risk of one diabetes-related end point was reduced by 12% and microvascular events were reduced by 25% compared with the diet-alone group. The results may actually have been better in the intensively treated group compared with the diet-only group if fewer patients in the latter group had crossed over to specific therapy.

In the UKPDS, both sulfonylureas and insulin were associated with a greater weight gain as well as more hypoglycemic episodes than metformin. Treatment with the latter agent resulted in a greater improvement in outcome than with sulfonylurea/insulin treatment. Patients treated with metformin as first-step therapy had

10

a decrease in diabetes-related death of 42% and a 32% reduction in any diabetes-related end points compared with the diet-alone group. These results suggest that metformin may provide benefits that drugs that increase insulin levels do not. Other agents, such as acarbose, pramlintide, exenatide, and sitagliptin, have not been evaluated in controlled clinical trials that examine their impact on microvascular and macrovascular disease.

Thus although reduction in overall CV events with glycemic control have not been dramatic, there is still good reason to lower blood glucose levels in diabetic patients. Reduction of microvascular events does occur and this will also help to correct some of the metabolic abnormalities of the diabetic metabolic syndrome. As emphasized, management of BP and lipid abnormalities is of great importance.

SELECTED READING

The Action to Control Cardiovascular Risk in Diabetes Study Group. Effects of intensive glucose lowering in type 2 diabetes. *N Engl J Med.* 2008;358:2545-2549.

The ADVANCE Collaborative Group. Intensive blood glucose control and vascular outcomes in patients with type 2 diabetes. *N Engl J Med.* 2008;358:2560-2572.

American Diabetes Association. Standards of medical care in diabetes. *Diabetes Care.* 2009;32(suppl 1):S13-S61.

American Diabetes Association. Physical activity/exercise and diabetes. *Diabetes Care.* 2004;27(suppl 1):S58-S62.

Bakris G, Molitch M, Hewkin A, et al; STAR Investigators. Differences in glucose tolerance between fixed-dose antihypertensive drug combinations in people with metabolic syndrome. *Diabetes Care.* 2006;29:2592-2597.

Blonde L, Klein EJ, Han J, et al. Interim analysis of the effects of exenatide treatment on A1C, weight and cardiovascular risk factors over 82 weeks in 314 overweight patients with type 2 diabetes. *Diabetes Obes Metab.* 2006;8:436-447.

Bolli GB, DiMarcho S, Park GD, Pramming S, Koivisto VA. Insulin analogues and their potential in the management of diabetes mellitus. *Diabetologia.* 1999;42:1151-1167.

Buse JB, Henry RR, Han J, Kim DD, Fineman MS, Baron AD; Exenatide-113 Clinical Study Group. Effects of exenatide (exendin-4) on glycemic control over 30 weeks in sulfonylurea treated patients with type 2 diabetes. *Diabetes Care*. 2004;27:2628-2635.

Buse JB; The ACCORD Study Group. Action to Control Cardiovascular Risk in Diabetes (ACCORD) Trial: design and methods. *Am J Cardiol*. 2007;99:S21-S31.

Canga N, De Irala J, Vara E, Duaso MJ, Ferrer A, Martinez-Gonzalez MA. Intervention study for smoking cessation in diabetic patients: a randomized controlled trial in both clinical and primary care setting. *Diabetes Care*. 2000;23:1455-1460.

Capes SE, Hunt D, Malmberg K, Gerstein HC. Stress hyperglycemia and increased risk of death after myocardial infarction in patients with and without diabetes: a systematic overview. *Lancet*. 2000;355:773-778.

Davidson MB, Peters AL. An overview of metformin in the treatment of type 2 diabetes mellitus. *Am J Med*. 1997;102:99-110.

DeFronzo RA, Ratner RE, Han J, et al. Effects of exenatide (exendin-4) on glycemic control and weight over 30 weeks in metformin-treated patients with type 2 diabetes. *Diabetes Care*. 2005;28:1092-1100.

The Diabetes Control and Complications Trial Research Group. The effect of intensive treatment of diabetes on the development and progression of long-term complications in insulin-dependent diabetes mellitus. *N Engl J Med*. 1993;329:977-986.

Dormandy JA, Charbonnel B, Eckland DJ, et al; PROactive investigators. Secondary prevention of macrovascular events in patients with type 2 diabetes in the PROactive Study (PROspective pioglitAzone Clinical Trial In macrovascular Events): a randomised controlled trial. *Lancet*. 2005;366(9493):1279-1289.

DREAM (Diabetes REduction Assessment with ramipril and rosiglitazone Medication) Trial Investigators; Gerstein HC, Yusuf S, Bosch J, et al. Effect of rosiglitazone on the frequency of diabetes in patients with impaired glucose tolerance or impaired fasting glucose: a randomised controlled trial. *Lancet*. 2006;368:1096-1105.

Duckworth W, Abraira C, Moritz T, et al; for the VADT Investigators. Glucose control and vascular complications in veterans with type 2 diabetes. *N Engl J Med*. 2009;360:129-139.

Home PD, Jones NP, Pocock SJ, et al; RECORD Study Group. Rosiglitazone RECORD study: glucose control outcomes at 18 months. *Diabet Med*. 2007;24:626-634.

Jacober SJ, Sowers JR. An update on perioperative management of diabetes. *Arch Intern Med*. 1999;159:2405-2411.

Khan KA, Govindarajan G, Whaley-Connell A, Sowers JR. Diabetic hypertension. *Heart Fail Clin*. 2006;2:25-36.

Lachin JM, Christophi CA, Edelstein SL, et al; DDK Research Group. Factors associated with diabetes onset during metformin versus placebo therapy in the diabetes prevention program. *Diabetes*. 2007;56:1153-1159.

McFarlane SI, Banerji M, Sowers JR. Insulin resistance and cardiovascular disease. *J Clin Endocrinol Metab*. 2001;86:713-718.

Nathan DM. Rosiglitazone and cardiotoxicity—weighing the evidence. *N Engl J Med*. 2007;357:64-67.

Nathan DM, Berkwits M. Trials that matter: rosiglitazone, ramipril, and the prevention of type 2 diabetes. *Ann Intern Med*. 2007;146:461-463.

Nissen SE, Wolski K. Effect of rosiglitazone on the risk of myocardial infarction and death from cardiovascular causes. *N Engl J Med*. 2007;356:1-15.

Psaty BM, Furberg CD. The record on rosiglitazone and the risk of myocardial infarction. *N Engl J Med*. 2007;357:67-69.

Ray KK, Seshasai SR, Wijesuriya S, et al. Effect of intensive control of glucose on cardiovascular outcomes and death in patients with diabetes mellitus: a meta-analysis of randomised controlled trials. *Lancet*. 2009;373:1765-1772.

Raz I, Hanefeld M, Xu L, et al; Sitagliptin Study 023 Group. Efficacy and safety of the dipeptidyl peptidase-4 inhibitor sitagliptin as monotherapy in patients with type 2 diabetes mellitus. *Diabetologia*. 2006;49:2564-2571.

UK Prospective Diabetes Study Group. Intensive blood-glucose control with sulphonylureas or insulin compared with conventional treatment and risk of complications in patients with type 2 diabetes (UKPDS 33). *Lancet*. 1998;352:837-853.

Uwaifo GI, Ratner RE. Differential effects of oral hypoglycemic agents on glucose control and cardiovascular risk. *Am J Cardiol*. 2007;99(4A):51B-67B.

Williamson DF, Thompson TJ, Thun M, Flanders D, Pamuk E, Byers T. Intentional weight loss mortality among overweight individuals with diabetes. *Diabetes Care*. 2000;23:1499-1504.

Zoungas S, de Galan BE, Ninomiya T; ADVANCE Collaborative Group. Combined effects of routine blood pressure lowering and intensive glucose control on macrovascular and microvascular outcomes in patients with type 2 diabetes: New results from the ADVANCE trial. *Diabetes Care*. 2009;32:2068-2074.

11 Risk Reduction in Special Populations

Treatment Considerations in Women

■ **Background**

Women are more susceptible to CVD following menopause for a number of reasons. LDL-cholesterol levels are often lower in premenopausal women than those in men, rising to higher levels after menopause. Triglyceride and LP(a) levels rise and HDL levels decrease after menopause. Low HDL cholesterol is a strong predictor of CHD in women as well as in men and, in the Lipids Research Clinics Follow-up Study, was second only to age as a predictor of CVD death. Trials of statins in secondary prevention of CVD, such as 4S and CARE, indicate that women benefit similarly to men. The CARE trial even suggests that they may benefit more as a result of their higher absolute risk if they have had a MI or stroke.

■ **Diabetes in Women**

Diabetes eliminates most of the protection normally afforded by female sex hormones in premenopausal women. Mortality rates from CHD are between three and seven times higher in diabetic women compared with nondiabetic women in contrast to the 2-fold to 4-fold increase in diabetic vs nondiabetic men.

CVD is the leading cause of death in women in the United States, accounting for 30% of all deaths. More than 225,000 women die annually from acute MI, and >85,000 women die from stroke. The numbers have decreased in recent years as a result of better treatment of hypertension and dyslipidemia. The incidence of CHD increases with age, and women >75 years of age constitute the most rapidly growing segment of our population. The mortality from CVD is greater in women than in men, as women typically have more risk factors (ie, systolic hypertension and glucose intolerance) than do men presenting with their initial MI or stroke. Thus the increase in CVD in women parallels the increasing incidence of both diabetes and hypertension.

Increasing obesity in adult women increases the risk for both diabetes and hypertension. Questionnaire data from the Nurses' Health Study cohort of 114,824 women reported that the risk for diabetes increased considerably when the BMI was >22 kg/m^2. Weight gain after the age of 18 years was strongly related to the risk for developing type 2 diabetes. In contrast, women who lost >5 kg from early adult life had a significantly reduced risk for development of diabetes. These data suggest that any weight gain in women during adulthood increases their risk of developing type 2 diabetes.

Women with diabetes are also more likely to die after an MI than women who do not have diabetes or men with or without diabetes. The risk of death from CHD in women with diabetes is more than three times that in nondiabetic women. As in men, an MI may be "silent" in diabetic women, ie, infarctions (even fatal ones) can occur with little or no chest pain only to be discovered at autopsy or in a routine ECG. Many risk factors contribute to the increase in CVD in diabetic women, including endothelial dysfunction, hypercoagulability, abnormalities of platelet function, dyslipidemia, and hypertension. Thus as for diabetic men, women with this disease should be treated with aspirin, have their LDL cholesterol lowered to <100 mg/dL, and their BP treated to a goal of <130/80-85 mm Hg. The ACCORD trial will include adequate numbers of women as well as ethnic minorities to determine if these groups also benefit from even more rigorous glycemic and BP control than currently recommended (see *Chapter 10*).

■ Role of HRT in Diabetic Women

Data have questioned whether diabetic postmenopausal women should receive HRT. There had been circumstantial evidence from the Postmenopausal Estrogen/Progestin Interventions (PEPI) trial that HRT would improve lipids in women who are not diabetic and who have not had prior CVD events. In a case-control study of

334 diabetic women, the use of postmenopausal estrogen replacement was not associated with an increased risk of CVD. However, there are reasons for concern about starting HRT in diabetic women. First, the risk of endometrial carcinoma is increased in diabetic women. Second, as noted repeatedly, persons who have diabetes but who do not have evidence of vascular disease may manifest the same risk for MI and stroke as nondiabetic persons who have already had such events. Accordingly, it would be anticipated that diabetic women would respond to HRT similarly to women with CVD, ie, as in the Heart and Estrogen/Progestin Replacement Study (HERS), where the risk of a CHD event was increased in women who received HRT. HRT should probably be limited to a short term (<1 year) in patients with annoying symptoms.

Treatment Considerations in Patients With Renal Disease

Control of both glycemia and BP is important in slowing the progression of renal disease in patients with either type 1 or type 2 diabetes. Systolic hypertension is a powerful promotor of renal disease progression in such patients. The rate of decline of renal function in patients with diabetic nephropathy is a continuous function of SBP levels down to approximately 125 mm Hg and DBP levels down to 70 to 75 mm Hg. One observational study showed that patients whose SBP was maintained <140 mm Hg did not display any deterioration in renal function. Conversely, those with SBP levels >140 mm Hg showed a substantial decline in renal function.

11

In a prospective interventional study of type 1 diabetic patients with hypertension, lowering mean arterial pressure from 143/96 to 130/84 mm Hg with β-blockers and diuretics slowed the decline in GFR by 77%. The Collaborative Study Group showed a 51% slower time to dialysis and doubling of serum creatinine among type 1 hypertensive diabetic patients who received an ACE inhibitor in addition to other agents compared with a regimen that did not include an ACE inhibitor. These differences could not be completely explained by significant differences in arterial BP. This advantage of

ACE inhibitors and ARBs in protecting renal function in diabetic patients, especially those with proteinuria, has been confirmed in longer-term studies in both type 1 and type 2 diabetic patients.

Patients with severe renal disease and nephrotic syndrome also appear to benefit from ACE and ARB therapy. Finally, it is clear from a number of long-term studies that persons with diabetes who achieve BP levels of ≤130/80 mm Hg have the slowest rates of decline in renal function. In a retrospective analysis of the Modified Dietary Protein in Renal Disease (MDRD) trial, patients who had >1 g/day of proteinuria, regardless of etiology, had slower rates of renal disease progression when the BP was <125/75 mm Hg. The results of AASK also suggest that the use of an ACE inhibitor–based program probably is beneficial in reducing overall morbidity and mortality in patients with nephropathy, especially in individuals with significant proteinuria. However, in this study, patients who achieved BP levels <130/80 mm Hg did not experience a better outcome than those with less rigid BP control. Thus, this trial did not confirm the need to reduce BP to levels <130/80 mm Hg in this population. As noted, however, the consensus is that lower levels of BP should be achieved in diabetic subjects than in the general hypertensive population.

The results of the RENAAL, IDNT, and IRMA 2 trials indicate that a regimen that includes the use of an ARB in type 2 diabetic patients with evidence of renal disease will slow the progression of renal disease and reduce proteinuria a significant degree compared with regimens that do not include an ARB.

Thus all diabetic patients with microalbuminuria should be receiving an ACE inhibitor or an ARB and should have their BP controlled to <130/80-85 mm Hg. This usually will require multiple medications, one of which should be a diuretic. If significant proteinuria (ie, ≥1 g) is present, BP should be treated to an even more rigorous goal (ie, 125/75 mm Hg), if at all possible. A reasonable guideline which, however, is not supported by good clinical data from clinical trials is to attempt to reduce BP to optimal levels of about 120/80 mm Hg in all patients consistent with few adverse effects.

SELECTED READINGS

Abu-Hamden DR, Sowers JR. Diabetes, dyslipidemia and renal disease in the elderly. *CVR&R*. 1998;2:60-64.

Bakris GL, Williams M, Dworkin L, et al for the National Kidney Foundation Hypertension and Diabetes Executive Committees Working Group. Preserving renal function in adults with hypertension and diabetes: a consensus approach. *Am J Kidney Dis*. 2000;36:645-661.

Kanaya AM, Grady D, Barrett-Connor E. Explaining the sex difference in coronary heart disease mortality among patients with type 2 diabetes: a meta-analysis. *Arch Intern Med*. 2002;162:1737-1745.

Kaseta JB, Skafar DF, Ram JL, Jacober SJ, Sowers JR. Cardiovascular disease in the diabetic woman. *J Clin Endocrinol Metab*. 1999;84:1835-1838.

McFarlane SI, Castro J, Kaur J, et al. Control of blood pressure and other cardiovascular risk fators at different practice settings: outcomes of care provided to diabetic women compared to men. *J Clin Hypertens*. 2005;7:73-80.

Natarajan S, Liao Y, Cao G, Lipsitz SR, McGee DL. Sex differences in risk for coronary heart disease mortality associated with diabetes and established coronary heart disease. *Arch Intern Med*. 2003;163:1735-1740.

Sowers JR, Neutel JM, Saunders E, et al; INCLUSIVE Investigators. Antihypertensive efficacy of irbesartan/HCTZ in men and women with the metabolic syndrome and type 2 diabetes. *J Clin Hypertens*. 2006;8:470-480.

11

12 Target Organs and Diabetes

Stroke in Diabetic Patients

Stroke is still the third leading cause of death in the United States. There are about 700,000 strokes annually and >4.5 million stroke survivors. Epidemiologic data indicate that there has been a leveling off of stroke-related mortality, but stroke and stroke death have decreased by >50% in the past 2 decades as the treatment of hypertension has improved. It has been suggested that high-risk or stroke-prone persons should be targeted for aggressive, preventive measures and specific interventions. Diabetes is an important and independent modifiable stroke-risk factor of increasing significance as our population ages and mortality from other causes decreases. Diabetic patients are not only more likely to suffer thrombotic strokes, but are also more likely to die, suffer permanent disability, and those that survive are more likely to have a second stroke than those without diabetes.

The worldwide incidence of stroke among patients with diabetes is more than three times that in the general population, with especially high risks in Scandinavian countries and the southeastern United States. Among Hawaiian Japanese men in the Honolulu Heart Program, the diabetic patients were at twice the risk for thromboembolic stroke as nondiabetics, independent of other factors known to predispose to stroke. In the Framingham Heart Study, people with glucose intolerance had double the risk for stroke compared with nondiabetics; the relative risk was greater in diabetic women compared with men, especially in the group 40 to 60 years of age.

Patients presenting with a stroke are more likely to have undiagnosed type 2 diabetes as well as serum glucose levels >180 mg/dL at 1 hour after a 50-g glucose load. Proteinuria is also a risk factor for stroke, both in people with impaired glucose tolerance and diabetes.

Blacks and Hispanics have a >2-fold increased incidence of stroke compared with white patients, perhaps reflecting the greater propensity for both diabetes and hypertension in these ethnic groups.

Both short-term and long-term mortality are increased in diabetic patients experiencing a stroke. The increased morbidity and mortality following a stroke correlates with glucose levels.

Hypertension is common in diabetic patients. In an 8-year observation of patients in the UKPDS, the increased risk of stroke in diabetic persons was strongly associated with the degree of BP elevation, particularly SBP elevation. Even diabetic patients with SBP between 125 and 142 mm Hg had twice as high a risk for stroke as persons with lower SBP.

■ Stroke Prevention in Diabetic Patients

As noted, data from the UKPDS reported a 44% relative risk reduction for stroke in the group whose BP was controlled (mean BP of 144/82 mm Hg) compared with the groups with poorer BP control (mean BP of 154 mm Hg). This 44% risk reduction was even greater than the 20% observed in diabetic patients in the SHEP. Better control of BP was a more significant factor in lowering risk of any diabetes-related end point than intensive blood glucose control.

The nitrendipine-based antihypertensive therapy trial (SYST-EUR multicenter trial) also demonstrated that an excess risk of stroke associated with diabetes was abolished by rigorous antihypertensive treatment of older patients with type 2 diabetes and isolated systolic hypertension. In diabetic patients in the Micro-Hope subanalysis of the HOPE study, there was a reduction of stroke by 33% with ACE inhibitor therapy superimposed on other antihypertensive drugs, antiplatelet therapy (primarily aspirin), lipid-lowering therapy (primarily HMG-CoA reductase inhibitor therapy), anticoagulants, and nitrates compared with therapy that did not include an ACE inhibitor.

The benefits of diuretic therapy as part of a regimen designed to reduce BP, especially SBP, were clearly established for the relatively large diabetic cohort in the

ALLHAT. Other studies have demonstrated the beneficial effects of ARBs, diuretic/ACE inhibitor combinations, and ACE inhibitor/CCB combinations in the primary and secondary preventions, respectively, of stroke in diabetic patients. In the PROGRESS study, recurrent stroke was reduced with an ACE inhibitor/diuretic combination but not with ACE inhibitor therapy alone.

■ Atrial Fibrillation/Anticoagulation

The observational data from the UKPDS also identified atrial fibrillation as an important risk factor for stroke in diabetic patients; diabetic patients between 35 and 74 years of age who had atrial fibrillation on an ECG were eight times more likely to suffer a stroke during the first 8 years of the study than those who were in sinus rhythm. In an 8-year population-based study of persons aged 35 to 74 years, 15.1% of diabetic patients with stroke had previously documented atrial fibrillation compared with 10.7% of those without diabetes.

Warfarin therapy has been shown to be associated with a two-thirds reduction in the risk of stroke when given for atrial fibrillation. The role of anticoagulants in the secondary prevention of stroke in patients with atrial fibrillation, especially in people with diabetes whose risk of cerebral hemorrhage appears to be less than those without diabetes, is of proven benefit. For primary prevention of stroke, patients with diabetes and atrial fibrillation should be on slightly reduced doses of warfarin in the absence of clear contraindications to maintain an international normalized ratio (INR) range of 2.0 to 3.0. If there are contraindications for warfarin, these patients should be maintained on aspirin therapy (81-325 mg/day).

■ Dyslipidemia

A number of prospective studies have shown a significant reduction in the risk of stroke with the use of lipid-lowering drugs in patients with increased risk for thromboembolic stroke, including people with diabetes. These studies include the 4S, CARE, the Medical Research Council/British Heart Foundation (MRC/BHF) HPS, and ASCOT. Recommendations from the ADA, as well as other agencies, note that statins are indicated in diabetics to achieve a goal LDL of <100 mg/dL for the primary prevention of stroke as well as MI. If a statin alone is ineffective in reducing LDL levels or in raising HDL levels, combination therapy with a fibrate may be indicated. Careful attention to reducing BP, lipid levels, and glucose levels in diabetic populations will be helpful in reducing the occurrence of carotid artery lesions, a frequent precursor of stroke.

■ **Summary**

The incidence and severity of stroke are increased in the diabetic patient. Stroke prevention, whether primary or secondary, has proven effective. Prevention measures include rigorous treatment of hypertension, antiplatelet and anticoagulant therapy, and the use of statin therapy. Lifestyle interventions include reduction of dietary salt and fat, smoking cessation, weight reduction, and limitation of alcohol consumption to no more than two drinks per day.

Heart Failure in Diabetes

There is an increased incidence of CHF in diabetes irrespective of coronary artery or hypertensive disease. This unique diabetic cardiac muscle disease is characterized by delayed diastolic relaxation, resulting from a direct effect of hyperglycemia, and altered insulin action on cardiac myocytes, a condition known as diabetic cardiomyopathy. Thus patients with type 2 diabetes have a high incidence of heart failure not only related to increased CHD and increased hypertensive disease, but also due to diabetic cardiomyopathy.

Framingham Heart Study data revealed a 4-fold greater incidence of CHF in diabetic men and an 8-fold increase in diabetic women compared with nondiabetic persons. Data from the Diabetes Mellitus Insulin-Glucose Infusion in Acute Myocardial Infarction (DIGAMI) trial indicate that CHF accounted for up to 66% of mortality among diabetic patients post-MI during the first year of follow-up. The high incidence of mortality following MI in diabetes is due, in part, to a higher incidence of post-MI CHF as well as arrhythmia-associated death.

Hypertensive cardiomyopathy is a major contributor to CHF in diabetic patients. After adjustment for age and weight, the relationship between increased hypertension and CHF remains.

Hyperglycemia contributes to CHF incidence in patients with diabetes, in part because of increased ischemic cardiomyopathy. The risk of CVD events, including CHF, rises >1% for every 1% increase in HbA_{1C}. Several trials have shown a trend in reduction of CVD events in diabetic patients with improved glycemic control. Dyslipidemia also contributes to ischemic cardiomyopathy and CVD, as previously discussed.

There is mounting evidence that diabetic cardiomyopathy is related in part to increased angiotensin II overexpression in diabetic hearts, and angiotensin II receptors (AT_1) are significantly upregulated in diabetic cardiomyocytes. Overexpression of the AT_1 receptor and elevated angiotensin II contributes to both increased fibrosis and apoptosis in diabetic hearts. Both elevated glucose and aldosterone have been shown to stimulate fibrosis and likely contribute significantly to development of CHF in diabetes. Blockade of the RAAS with an ACE inhibitor, an ARB, an α-blocker/β-blocker, or a β-blocker may offer a physiologically appropriate approach to preventing and treating CHF in diabetic patients.

Sudden Cardiac Death and Diabetes

Diabetes is associated with a substantial increase in the incidence of sudden cardiac death. The proposed mechanisms for sudden death in diabetic patients include abnormalities of the autonomic nervous system. These abnormalities include enhanced sympathetic activity and diminished parasympathetic activity. ECG abnormalities predisposing to fatal ventricular arrhythmias, such as QTc prolongation and increased QTc dispersion, are found with increased frequency in both type 1 and type 2 DM. Holter monitoring in diabetic patients has shown that the diurnal and nocturnal levels of low frequency/ high frequency heart rates, an index of parasympathetic to sympathetic balance, are significantly reduced in persons with diabetic autonomic neuropathy. The normal day-to-night modulation of QT/RR relation is often altered, with a reversed day-night pattern and an increased nocturnal QT-rate dependence. Many individuals with the cardio-metabolic syndrome and type 2 diabetes demonstrate reduced RR variability indicative of altered autonomic control. Persons with the cardiometabolic syndrome are at increased risk for sudden death, up to two to three times more frequently than those with normal glucose metabolism. Correction of glycemia, hypertension, and lipid levels, as well as maintaining adequate levels of potassium, magnesium, and chromium intake, may be helpful in reducing the occurrence of sudden death in this population.

■ Current Control of CVD Risk Factors in Diabetic Patients

In a retrospective chart-review analysis, only 25% to 30% of diabetic patients were treated to goal BP levels of 130/80 mm Hg. Inadequate treatment largely reflected lack of SBP control. As reviewed in *Chapter 6*, uncertainly about achievable levels of BP, especially in older patients, may account for the less than adequate BP control in many diabetic patients. Only 25% to 30% of surveyed patients had achieved HbA_{1C} <7% and 50% still had HbA_{1C} >8%. In another analysis, 35% of diabetic subjects had levels of LDL cholesterol <100 mg/dL, but one third had LDL cholesterol levels >130 mg/dL. Data indicate that only 50% of eligible diabetic patients are treated with aspirin. Despite the particularly high risk of CVD among women with diabetes, they are not treated aggressively with lipid therapy and fewer women than men are currently receiving aspirin.

SELECTED READING

Davis TM, Millns H, Stratton IM, Holman RR, Turner RC. Risk factors for stroke in type 2 diabetes mellitus: United Kingdom Prospective Diabetes Study (UKPDS) 29. *Arch Intern Med*. 1999;159:1097-1103.

Effects of ramipril on cardiovascular and microvascular outcomes in people with diabetes mellitus: results of the HOPE study and MICRO-HOPE substudy. Heart Outcomes Prevention Evaluation Study Investigators. *Lancet*. 2000;355:253-259.

Fagan TC, Sowers J. Type 2 diabetes mellitus: greater cardiovascular risks and greater benefits of therapy. *Arch Intern Med*. 1999;159:1033-1034.

Gustafsson I, Hildebrandt P. Early failure of the diabetic heart. *Diabetes Care*. 2001;24:3-4.

Haffner SM. Coronary heart disease in patients with diabetes. *N Engl J Med*. 2000;342:1040-1042.

Kurukulasuriya LR, Govindarajan G, Sowers J. Stroke prevention in diabetes and obesity. *Expert Rev Cardiovasc Ther*. 2006;4:487-502.

Lindholm LH, Ibsen H, Dahlof B, et al; LIFE Study Group. Cardiovascular morbidity and mortality in patients with diabetes in the Losartan Intervention For Endpoint reduction in hypertension study (LIFE): a randomised trial against atenolol. *Lancet*. 2002;359:1004-1010.

McFarlane SI, Sica DA, Sowers JR. Stroke in patients with diabetes and hypertension. *J Clin Hypertens*. 2005;7:286-292.

PROGRESS Collaborative Group. Randomised trial of a perindopril-based blood-pressure-lowering regimen among 6,105 individuals with previous stroke or transient ischaemic attack. *Lancet*. 2001;358:1033-1041.

Sacco RL. Reducing the risk of stroke in diabetes: what have we learned that is new? *Diabetes Obes Metab*. 2002;4(suppl 1):S27-S34.

Sowers JR. Hypertension, angiotensin II, and oxidative stress. *N Engl J Med*. 2002;346:1999-2001.

Sowers JR, Neutel JM, Saunders E, et al; INCLUSIVE Investigators. Antihypertensive efficacy of irbesartan/HCTZ in men and women with the metabolic syndrome and type 2 diabetes. *J Clin Hypertens (Greenwich)*. 2006;8:470-480.

Valensi PE, Johnson NB, Maison-Blanche P, Extramania F, Motte G, Coumel P. Influence of cardiac autonomic neuropathy on heart rate dependence of ventricular repolarization in diabetic patients. *Diabetes Care*. 2002;25:918-923.

12

13 Summary of Cardiovascular Disease Reduction in Diabetic Patients

CVD accounts for up to 80% of premature mortal events in persons with diabetes. Thus all strategies to reduce this risk should be optimized in these persons. All patients who tolerate aspirin should receive a minimum aspirin dose of 81 mg/day up to one adult aspirin 325 mg/day. Further, since diabetic patients without evidence of vascular disease have almost the same CVD risk as nondiabetics who have already had an MI or stroke, their LDL cholesterol should be lowered at least to <100 mg/dL or, if at all possible, to <70 mg/dL. Importantly, BP should be lowered, if necessary, and maintained as close as possible to optimal levels of about 120/80 mm Hg. If they can tolerate an ACE inhibitor or an ARB, they should receive one of these agents (usually in addition to a low-dose diuretic). A β-blocker may also be appropriate in some cases. The addition of a calcium antagonist may be necessary to lower BP to <130/80-85 mm Hg. The use of an ARB may have some advantages over an ACE inhibitor—less concern for the rare case of angioedema or a cough. Use of RAAS inhibitors is especially compelling in those diabetic patients with proteinuria.

Optimal glycemic control should be attempted, even though this strategy has not been proven consistently to lower CVD risk. It is critical to engage diabetic patients in hygienic measures, including weight reduction, moderate exercise, discontinuation of smoking, and moderation of alcohol intake. A comprehensive guide to primary prevention of CVD in diabetics is presented in **Table 13.1**.

Summary

The management of diabetes has evolved significantly since the discovery of insulin and the realization

TABLE 13.1 — Recommendations for Primary Prevention of CVD in People With Diabetes

Weight

- Structured programs that emphasize lifestyle changes such as reduced fat (<30% of daily energy) and total energy intake and increased regular physical activity, along with regular participant contact, can produce long-term weight loss on the order of 5% to 7% of starting weight, with improvement in BP
- For individuals with elevated plasma triglycerides and reduced HDL cholesterol, improved glycemic control, moderate weight loss (5% to 7% of starting weight), dietary saturated fat restriction, increased physical activity, and modest replacement of dietary carbohydrate (5% to 7%) by either monounsaturated or polyunsaturated fats may be beneficial
- Medical nutrition therapy:
  - To achieve reductions in LDL cholesterol:
    - Saturated fats should be <7% of energy intake
    - Dietary cholesterol intake should be <200 mg/d
    - Intake of trans unsaturated fatty acids should be <1% of energy intake
  - Total energy intake should be adjusted to achieve body-weight goals
  - Total dietary fat intake should be moderated (25% 35% of total calories) and should consist mainly of monounsaturated or polyunsaturated fat
  - Ample intake of dietary fiber ($\geq$14 g per 1000 calories consumed) may be of benefit
  - If individuals choose to drink alcohol, daily intake should be limited to one drink for adult women and two drinks for adult men (one drink is defined as a 12-oz beer, a 4-oz glass of wine, or a 1.5-oz glass of distilled spirits). Alcohol ingestion increases caloric intake and should be minimized when weight loss is the goal. Individuals with elevated plasma triglyceride levels should limit alcohol intake, because intake may exacerbate hypertriglyceridemia
  - In both normotensive and hypertensive individuals, a reduction in sodium intake may lower BP. The goal should be to reduce sodium intake to 1200-2300 mg/d, equivalent to 3000-6000 mg/d of sodium chloride

Physical Activity

- To improve glycemic control, assist with weight loss or maintenance, and reduce risk of CVD, at least 150

Continued

minutes of moderate-intensity aerobic physical activity or at least 90 minutes of more vigorous aerobic exercise per week is recommended. Brisk walking is especially recommended. Physical activity should be distributed over at least 3 days per week, with no >2 consecutive days without physical activity

Blood Pressure

- BP should be measured at every routine diabetes visit. Patients found to have SBP ≥130 mm Hg or DBP ≥80 mm Hg should have BP confirmed on a separate day
- Patients with diabetes should be treated to an SBP <130 mm Hg and a DBP <80 mm Hg, if at all possible
- Patients with an SBP of 130-139 mm Hg or a DBP of 80-89 mm Hg should initiate lifestyle modification alone (weight control, increased physical activity, alcohol moderation, sodium reduction, and emphasis on increased consumption of fresh fruits, vegetables, and low-fat dairy products) for a maximum of 1-2 months. If after these efforts targets are not achieved, treatment with pharmacological agents should be initiated
- Patients with hypertension (SBP ≥140 mm Hg or DBP ≥90 mm Hg) should receive drug therapy in addition to lifestyle and behavioral therapy
- All patients with diabetes and hypertension should be treated with a regimen that includes either an ACE inhibitor or an ARB. The use of a diuretic is also necessary in most cases to achieve goal BP. If one class is not tolerated, the other should be substituted. Other drug classes demonstrated to reduce CVD events in patients with diabetes (β-blockers and CCBs) should be added as needed to achieve BP targets
- If ACE inhibitors, ARBs, or diuretics are used, renal function and serum potassium levels should be monitored within the first 3 months. If stable, follow-up could occur every 6 months thereafter
- Multiple-drug therapy is generally required to achieve BP targets
- In elderly hypertensive patients, BP should be lowered gradually to avoid complications
- Orthostatic measurement of BP should be performed in people with diabetes and hypertension when clinically indicated, especially in the elderly
- Patients not achieving target BP despite multiple-drug therapy should be referred to a physician specializing in the care of patients with hypertension

13

Continued

TABLE 13.1 — *Continued*

Lipids

- In adult patients, test for lipid disorders at least annually and more often if needed to achieve goals. In adults <40 yo with relatively normal lipid values (LDL cholesterol <100 mg/dL, HDL cholesterol >50 mg/dL, and triglycerides <150 mg/dL), lipid assessments may be repeated every 2 years
- Lifestyle modifications deserve primary emphasis in all diabetic individuals. Patients should focus on the reduction of saturated fat and cholesterol intake, weight loss (if indicated), and increases in dietary fiber and physical activity. These lifestyle changes have been shown to improve the lipid profile in patients with diabetes
- In individuals with diabetes who are >40 yo without overt CVD but with one or more major CVD risk factors, the primary goal is an LDL level <100 mg/dL. If LDL-lowering drugs are used, a reduction of at least 30% to 40% in LDL levels should be obtained. If baseline LDL is <100 mg/dL, statin therapy should be initiated based on risk factor assessment and clinical judgment. Major risk factors in this category include cigarette smoking, hypertension (BP >140/90 mm Hg or use of antihypertensive medication), low HDL (<40 mg/dL), and family history of premature CHD (CHD in male first-degree relative ≤55 yo; CHD in female first-degree relative ≤65 yo)
- In individuals with diabetes who are <40 yo without overt CVD but who are estimated to be at increased risk of CVD either by clinical judgment or by risk calculator, the LDL goal is <100 mg/dL, and LDL-lowering drugs should be considered if lifestyle changes do not achieve the goal
- The ADA suggests lowering triglycerides to <150 mg/dL and raising HDL levels to >40 mg/dL. In women, an HDL goal 10 mg/dL higher (>50 mg/dL) should be considered
- Combination therapy of LDL-lowering drugs (eg, statins) and fibrates or niacin may be necessary to achieve lipid targets, but this has not been evaluated in outcome studies for either CVD event reduction or safety

Tobacco

- All patients with diabetes should be asked about tobacco use status at every visit
- Every tobacco user should be advised to quit
- The tobacco user's willingness to quit should be assessed

Continued

- The patient can be assisted by counseling and by developing a plan to quit
- Follow-up, referral to special programs, or pharmacotherapy (including nicotine replacement and bupropion) should be incorporated as needed

Antiplatelet Agents
- Aspirin therapy (81-162 mg/d) should be recommended as a primary prevention strategy in people with diabetes at increased CV risk, including those who are >40 yo or who have additional risk factors (family history of CVD, hypertension, smoking, dyslipidemia, or albuminuria)
- People with aspirin allergy, bleeding tendency, existing anticoagulant therapy, recent GI bleeding, and clinically active hepatic disease are not candidates for aspirin therapy. Other antiplatelet agents may be a reasonable alternative for patients at high risk
- Aspirin therapy should not be recommended for patients <21 yo because of the increased risk of Reye's syndrome associated with aspirin use in this population. People <30 yo have not been studied

Glycemic Control
- The A1C goal for patients in general is <7%
- The A1C goal for the individual patient is an A1C as close to normal (<6%) as possible, without causing significant hypoglycemia

Type 1 Diabetes
- At the present time, all of the recommendations listed above for patients with type 2 diabetes appear appropriate for those with type 1 diabetes as well

Adapted from: Buse JB, et al. *Diabetes Care.* 2007;30:162-172.

that correcting blood glucose abnormalities could slow down or prevent progression of kidney disease, retinopathy, and CVD. During the past 50 years, widespread efforts have been made to regulate blood glucose levels. These initially involved the manipulation of insulin dosage and nutritional interventions. Regimens were complicated, diets were difficult to follow, and insulin reactions were common.

With the discovery that diabetes is part of a complex metabolic syndrome and that insulin resistance plays a major role in the eventual development of diabetes in a majority of patients, a new approach was undertaken. New oral hypoglycemic drugs were marketed. Some of these increased the secretion of insulin; others helped to increase insulin utilization. With the introduction of more effective therapies and less dependence on rigid diets that required careful selections of components of various food groups, management improved. Longevity, both in the insulin-dependent type 1 diabetic and the much more common type 2 diabetic, increased significantly.

In recent years, it has become evident that most of the morbidity/mortality in diabetics is not related to diabetic microvascular events (ie, retinopathy and nephropathy). Although emphasis should still be placed on the prevention of these serious complications, the new paradigm suggests strongly that in the diabetic patient more attention must be placed on the prevention or management of other risk factors. Glycemic control is important, but control of elevated BP, lipid abnormalities, and smoking habits may be more important. These strategies have been shown to improve microvascular outcome, especially nephropathy, as well as reduce macrovascular disease in patients with both type 1 and type 2 diabetes.

In the *Clinical Management of Cardiovascular Risk Factors in Diabetes*, a review and update not only of the lifestyle management components of the diabetic patient, but of other risk factors that may play an even more important role in the outcome of these patients, is presented. Until recent years, little attention has been paid to these important factors:

- A majority of patients with diabetes and hypertension remain untreated and have not reached goal BP levels <130/80-85 mm Hg.
- A majority of diabetic patients, who should be considered high-risk individuals for CVD and essentially in the same category as nondiabetics who have already experienced a CV episode, have not been treated adequately with regard to the management of lipid disorders. In addition, efforts should be made to decrease triglyceride levels to <150 mg/dL and to raise HDL levels to >45 mg/dL if they are low. Most guidelines indicate that LDL levels should be treated to <70 mg/dL.
- Although the exact dose of aspirin is controversial, all diabetic patients should receive a minimum of

81 mg aspirin unless they have absolute contrain-dications, such as bleeding diathesis, or in patients ≤18 years of age due to a propensity of this age group to develop Reye disease.

The future of patients with type 2 diabetes, patients who now number >15 million in the United States, has been dramatically improved. This has occurred by paying more attention to CV risk factors in addition to blood sugar abnormalities. Much more can be done to prolong the lives of diabetics and importantly to decrease mortality from renal as well as CV complications.

Clinical Management of Cardiovascular Risk Factors in Diabetes has tried to outline the reasons for a multifaceted approach to the treatment of diabetes. The evolution of the management of diabetes has followed that of the treatment of hypertension. Initially, only symptomatic or severe type 1 diabetics were treated. Malignant hypertension was treated first and, as data were collected from the clinical trials, less severe hypertension was treated. Today, lowering BP in people with stage I disease (140-160/90-100 mm Hg) even without evidence of renal or cardiac disease is justified based on results of randomized clinical trials. Similarly, there are now enough studies in diabetic patients to justify a more aggressive approach to managing CV risk factors in this population, even in patients without evidence of CVD. Nevertheless, <5% of diabetic patients in the United States have their BP, LDL cholesterol, and glycemia treated to target goals of <130/80 mm Hg, <70 mg/dL, and an HbA_{1C} <7%, respectively.

As noted elsewhere in this book, management need not be complicated, expensive, or involved. Complicated procedures or frequent doctor visits may not be necessary. Most patients can modify their lifestyle and adhere to therapy for lowering BP and correct at least most of the lipid abnormalities as well as their blood glucose levels without turning their households into diet kitchens or radically changing their life.

13

Cooper SA, Whaley-Connell A, Habibi J, et al. Renin-angiotensin-aldo-sterone system and oxidative stress in cardiovascular insulin resistance. *Am J Physiol Heart Circ Physiol.* 2007;293:H2009-H2023.

Hayden MR, Sowers JR. Redox imbalance in diabetes. *Antioxid Redox Signal.* 2007;9:865-867.

Manrique CM, Lastra G, Palmer J, Stump CS, Sowers JR. Hyperten-sion–a treatable component of the cardiometabolic syndrome: chal-lenges for the primary care physician. *J Clin Hypertens (Greenwich).* 2006;8(1 suppl 1):12-20.

McFarlane SI, Castro J, Kaur J, et al. Control of blood pressure and other cardiovascular risk factors at different practice settings: outcomes of care provided to diabetic women compared to men. *J Clin Hypertens (Greenwich).* 2005;7:73-80.

Moser M, Ross H. The treatment of hypertension in diabetic patients. *Diabetes Care.* 1993;16:542-547.

Sowers JR. Treatment of hypertension in patients with diabetes. *Arch Intern Med.* 2004;164:1850-1857.

Stump CS, Hamilton MT, Sowers JR. Effect of antihypertensive agents on the development of type 2 diabetes mellitus. *Mayo Clin Proc.* 2006;81:796-806.

14

Abbreviations/Acronyms

4S	Scandinavian Simvastatin Survival Study
AASK	African American Study of Kidney Disease and Hypertension
ABCD	Appropriate Blood Pressure Control in Diabetes [study]
ACCOMPLISH	Avoiding Cardiovascular Events Through Combination Therapy in Patient Living With Systolic Hypertension [study]
ACCORD	Action to Control Cardiovascular Risk in Diabetes [study]
ACE	angiotensin-converting enzyme
ADA	American Diabetes Association
ADVANCE	Action in Diabetes and Vascular Disease: Preterax and Diamicron Modified Release Control Evaluation [study]
AE	adverse event
AFCAPS	Air Force Coronary Atherosclerosis Prevention Study
AHA	American Heart Association
AI	angiotensin 1
AII	angiotensin II
ALLAY	Aliskiren Left Ventricular Assessment of Hypertrophy [study]
ALLHAT	Antihypertensive and Lipid-Lowering Treatment to Prevent Heart Attack Trial
ALOFT	Aliskiren Observation of Heart Failure Treatment [study]
ANBP	Australian National Blood Pressure
ARB	angiotensin II receptor blocker
ARR	absolute risk reduction
ASCOT	Anglo-Scandinavian Cardiac Outcomes Trial
ASCOT-BPLA	Anglo-Scandinavian Cardiac Outcomes Trial–blood-pressure–lowering arm
ASCOT-LLA	Anglo-Scandinavian Cardiac Outcomes Trial–lipid-lowering arm

14

ASTEROID	Study to Evaluate the Effect of Rosuvastatin on Intravascular Ultrasound-Derived Coronary Atheroma Burden
ATP	Adult Treatment Panel
AT1R	angiotensin II type 1 receptor
AVOID	Aliskiren in the Evaluation of Proteinuria in Diabetes [study]
BHF	British Heart Foundation
bid	twice daily
BMI	body mass index
BP	blood pressure
CABG	coronary artery bypass grafting
CAPPP	Captopril Prevention Project [study]
CARDS	Collaborative Atorvastatin Diabetes Study
CARE	Cholesterol and Recurrent Events [study]
CCB	calcium channel blocker
CHARM	Candesartan in Heart Failure—Assessment of Reduction in Mortality and Morbidity
CHD	coronary heart disease
CHF	congestive heart failure
CI	confidence interval
CKD	chronic kidney disease
CPK	creatine phosphokinase
CRP	C-reactive protein
CV	cardiovascular
CVD	cardiovascular disease
DAIS	Diabetes Atherosclerosis Intervention Study
DASH	Dietary Approaches to Stop Hypertension [study]
DBP	diastolic blood pressure
DCCT	Diabetes Control and Complications Trial
DIGAMI	Diabetes Mellitus Insulin-Glucose Infusion in Acute Myocardial Infarction [study]
DM	diabetes mellitus
DPP	Diabetes Prevention Program
DPP-IV	dipeptidyl peptidase IV
DREAM	Diabetes Reduction Assessment With Ramipril and Rosiglitazone Medication [study]
ECG	electrocardiogram
ER	extended release
ESRD	end-stage renal disease
ET-1	endothelin-1
ETDRS	Early Treatment Diabetic Retinopathy Study

EUCLID	EURODIAB Controlled Trial of Lisinopril in Insulin-Dependent Diabetes Mellitus
EWPHE	European Working Party on High Blood Pressure in the Elderly
EXCEL	Expanded Clinical Evaluation of Lovastatin [study]
FACET	Fosinopril vs Amlodipine Cardiovascular Event Trial
FBG	fasting blood glucose
FDA	Food and Drug Administration
FFA	free fatty acid
FIELD	Fenofibrate Intervention and Event Lowering in Diabetes [study]
g	gram
GDM	gestational diabetes mellitus
GEMINI	Glycemic Effects in Diabetic Mellitus: Carvedilol-Metoprolol Comparison in Hypertensives [study]
GFR	glomerular filtration rate
GI	gastrointestinal
GLP-1	glucagonlike peptide-1
h	hour(s)
HAPPHY	Heart Attack Primary Prevention in Hypertension
HbA_{1C}	glycosylated hemoglobin
HCTZ	hydrochlorothiazide
HCV	hepatitis C virus
HDFP	Hypertension Detection Follow-up Program
HDL-c	high-density lipoprotein cholesterol
HERS	Heart and Estrogen/Progestin Replacement Study
HMG-CoA	3-hydroxy-3-methylglutaryl coenzyme A
HOPE	Heart Outcomes Prevention Evaluation
HOPE-TOO	Heart Outcomes Prevention Evaluation— The Ongoing Outcomes
HOT	Hypertension Optimal Treatment [study]
HPS	Heart Protection Study
HR	heart risk
HRT	hormone replacement therapy
IDF	International Diabetes Federation
IDL	intermediate-density lipoprotein
IDNT	Irbesartan Diabetic Nephropathy Trial
IFG	impaired fasting glucose
IGT	impaired glucose tolerance

14

IL	interleukin
INR	international normalized ratio
INSIGHT	International Nifedipine Gastrointestinal Therapeutic System Study Intervention as a Goal for Hypertension
INVEST	International Verapamil SR/Trandolapril Study
IRAS	Insulin Resistance Atherosclerosis Study
IRMA 2	Irbesartan Microalbuminuria Type 2 Diabetes Mellitus in Hypertension Patients Trial
ISH	isolated systolic hypertension
ITT	intention-to-treat
IVUS	intravascular ultrasound
JNC	Joint National Committee
kcal	kilogram calorie
lb	pound(s)
LDL-c	low-density lipoprotein cholesterol
LIFE	Losartan Intervention for Endpoint Reduction in Hypertension [study]
LIPID	Long-Term Intervention With Pravastatin in Ischaemic Disease [study]
Lp(a)	lipoprotein (a)
LS	least square
LVH	left ventricular hypertrophy
MDRD	Modified Dietary Protein in Renal Disease [study]
MI	myocardial infarction
min	minute(s)
MICRO-HOPE	Heart Outcomes Prevention Evaluation and Microalbuminuria, Cardiovascular, and Renal Outcomes [study]
MRC	Medical Research Council
MRFIT	Multiple Risk Factor Intervention Trial
n, N	number
NADPH	National Health and Nutrition Examination Survey
NCEP	National Cholesterol Education Program
NG	normoglycemic
NHANES	National Health and Nutrition Examination Survey
NHBLI	National Heart, Lung, and Blood Institute
NHES	National Health Examination Survey
NIH	National Institutes of Health

NO	nitric oxide
NOD	new-onset diabetes
NORDIL	Nordic Diltiazem [study]
OGTT	oral glucose tolerance test
ONTARGET	Ongoing Telmisartan Alone or in Combination With Ramipril Global Endpoint Trial
OR	odds ratio
PAI-1	plasminogen-activator inhibitor type 1
PEPI	Postmenopausal Estrogen/Progestin Interventions [study]
PROACTIVE	Prospective Pioglitazone Clinical Trial in Macrovascular Events
qd	every day
qhs	at bedtime
qpm	each evening
PROGRESS	Perindopril Protection Against Recurrent Stroke Study
RAS	renin-angiotensin system
RAAS	rennin-angiotensin-aldosterone system
RC	referred care
RDA	recommended daily allowance
RECORD	Rosiglitazone Evaluated for Cardiac Outcomes and Regulation of Glycaemia in Diabetes [study]
REGRESS	Regression Grown Evaluation Statin Study
RENAAL	Reduction of Endpoints in Noninsulin Dependent Diabetes Mellitus With an Angiotensin II Antagonist, Losartan [study]
ROS	reactive oxygen species
RR	relative risk
RRR	relative risk reduction
SANDS	Stop Atherosclerosis in Native Diabetics Study
SBP	systolic blood pressure
SC	stepped care
SCD	sudden cardiac death
SCOPE	Study on Cognition and Prognosis in the Elderly
SE	standard error of measurement
sec	second(s)
SHEP	Systolic Hypertension in the Elderly Program

14

STOP	Swedish Trial in Older Patients With Hypertension
SYST-EUR	Systolic Hypertension Trial in Europe
TexCAPS	Texas Coronary Atherosclerosis Prevention Study
TG	triglyceride
TGF-β	transforming growth factor-beta
tid	three times a day
TLC	therapeutic lifestyle changes
TNF-α	tumor necrosis factor-alpha
TOD	target-organ disease
TOMHS	Treatment of Mild Hypertension Study
tPA	tissue-type plasminogen activator
UK	United Kingdom
UKPDS	United Kingdom Prospective Diabetes Study
VA	Veterans Administration
VADT	Veterans Affairs Diabetes Trial
VA-HIT	Veterans Affairs High-Density Lipoprotein Cholesterol Intervention Trial
VALUE	Valsartan Antihypertensive Long-term Use Evaluation [study]
VLDL	very low-density lipoprotein
WHO	World Health Organization
wk	week(s)
WOSCOPS	West of Scotland Coronary Prevention Study
y	year
yo	years old

INDEX

Note: Page numbers in *italics* indicate figures.
Page numbers followed by a "t" indicate tables.
Clinical trials and studies are indexed under the acronym of the name;
cross-references are provided from the full name.

15

273

15

15

15

15

15

283

15

285

15

288

15

15

15

15

15

15

15

15